Lose Weight Naturally

LOSE WEIGHT NATURALLY

by Mark Bricklin
Executive Editor, Prevention® Magazine

Sharon Faelten,
Research Associate

Rodale Press 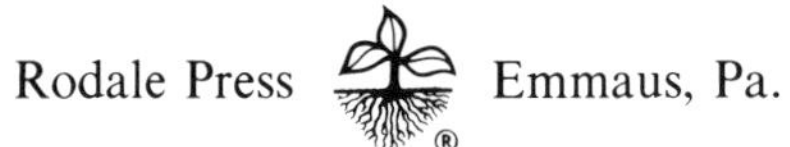 Emmaus, Pa.

Printed in the United States of America on recycled paper, containing a high percentage of de-inked fiber.

Library of Congress Cataloging in Publication Data

Mark Bricklin.
Lose weight naturally.

Includes index.
1. Reducing diets. 2. Reducing. I. Title.
RM222.2.B77 613.2′5 79-10873
ISBN 0-87857-252-X hardcover

6 8 10 9 7 5 hardcover

Table of Contents

Introduction

Until recently, I never thought I'd write a book on dieting.

Which is kind of strange, considering I'm a health writer and that overweight is probably the most common health problem in the United States today.

The reason, very simply, is that until this year, I was convinced there is no point in telling people how to reduce. I knew from personal experience, and that of many friends, that losing weight is easy. But gaining it back is easier. Much easier.

When I was around 30, I looked at a photograph taken of me in a bathing suit, bending over in a wading pool as I played with my daughter. I looked like Santa Claus, with all the toys stuffed in my gut instead of carried over my back. From the chest up, I looked as if I still weighed from 150 to 155 pounds — my weight before I'd been married. But from the chest down, I looked like about 195.

Naturally, I went on a diet.

It lasted almost three months and had me in a constant state of tension. And it didn't make me feel very good about myself — or about dieting in general — when I eventually went off the diet and quickly gained back almost everything I had so painfully lost.

What happened to me was discouraging, but not very unusual, it turned out. Almost everyone I talked to had lost at least 20 pounds at some point and then gained back anywhere from 18 to 25. The whole dieting thing made no sense to me. It was as if a man who is terribly tense and overworked were to say to himself, "This is no way to live! I've got to relax!" So he takes a lovely, two-week vacation on a quiet beach. One week and six days later, he feels as mellow as the Maharishi. But as soon as the return flight lands in at the airport, his nerves start racing again, and a week later, after scrambling like crazy to catch up on his work, he needs a vacation more than ever.

What our nervous friend really needs, of course, is not a vacation. What he needs is a new life-style. More basically, he needs to learn some techniques that will enable him to relax every day of his life.

Likewise, what the overweight person needs is not a diet, but some basic behavioral tools that will give him the wherewithal to become slender and *stay* that way — permanently.

Of course, I wouldn't be writing this now if I hadn't found those tools for myself.

In April of last year, I weighed 177. By July, I was down to 153, less than I've weighed in a dozen years. And now, in winter, I'm still down there, at about 150, with no pain or strain. That's what made me decide to share these tools with others.

Understand, I didn't invent these tools. I may have polished a few here and there, but basically they were invented and refined by doctors — mostly psychologists. You might say I purchased a set for myself, paying the price of perhaps four or five hours of reading and study. Over a period of months, I applied what I had learned — and learned a lot more in the process. And one of the things I eventually realized is that most, if not all, of the available literature on these new tools for reducing is too complicated and too demanding for the average person to put into action. Probably the reason for that is that these programs are generally conducted in face-to-face workshops or counseling sessions, in which it's much easier to explain things than in a book. Somehow, when the experts get to translating their ideas from the workshop setting to the printed page, too much of the message gets lost.

Keeping that in mind, I have attempted in this book to be as explicit as possible, anticipating problems and questions and repeating the basic points several times — just as if we were in a classroom setting. That's crucial, I think, because what we're doing here is not just handing out some simple instructions. Rather, we're presenting principles and techniques that need to be really understood and then applied in your own life — just as if you were learning how to fly an airplane or sell insurance. You can't learn to do things like that by reading instruction sheets, no matter how closely you follow them.

And neither will you learn how to lose weight and keep it off without learning the principles and *applying* the techniques that we'll present here.

As a final note before we begin, let me say that the reason I am so enthusiastic about this approach is not because it enabled me to reduce my waist size from 36 to 31. I'd come close to doing that before. The great thing about this approach is that I've been staying at that size for some time now, and my old pants still look like clown suits on me. Significantly, in these last months, I've been under considerable stress — not the least of which was writing this book. In fact, many times I've forgotten everything I know and gorged myself like I used to do in the old days. The difference has been that these incidents no longer bother me, no longer make me feel like I have no control over my appetite, no longer make me feel disgusted with myself. I accept them in a very neutral kind of way, knowing that in the long run they have very little significance, and that it will be easy to compensate for their excess. They are no more important or threatening than the "bumps" you often hit in plane travel: they may jar you or even upset you a little, but the experienced traveler knows they're nothing to worry about.

Just as an unexpected updraft or downdraft is neither going to send your airplane into orbit nor hurl it six miles down to the ground, *the inevitable bumps that you'll hit on your eating program will have no effect whatsoever on whether or not you reach your destination.* That's something you should know before you embark on your weight-control program. In fact, the confidence of knowing that the bumps are just bumps and not catastrophes will — perhaps more than anything else — help insure that your voyage is a success.

1

Get Ready for Something New

The first question everyone asks about a new diet plan is "How is this diet different? Why is it going to succeed when all the other diets I've tried have failed?"

Those are perfectly legitimate questions, and I want to answer them immediately. But I'm going to do that by making nine statements about weight reduction and ask you to read each of them and decide which are true and which false. *Please think carefully before answering.*

1. **My problem is that I need to lose weight — 20 or 30 or 50 or however many pounds.**
2. **My appetite is ungovernable — I just naturally want to gorge myself.**
3. **When you're following a diet, there's no substitute for willpower.**
4. **To follow a diet successfully, you need a special eating plan and special low-calorie meals. Or at least, they're a big help.**
5. **Three pounds a week is about the minimum loss that a good diet should produce.**
6. **In general, it's a good idea for the reducer to avoid such starchy, high-carbohydrate foods as bread, potatoes, beans, rice, and spaghetti.**

7. Fact: To burn up the calories in one piece of pie a la mode, you would have to do 50 push-ups, 100 deep knee bends, 200 sit-ups, and then run around the block half a dozen times! So exercise isn't really that important in reducing. It just isn't realistic.

8. It's good to weigh yourself every day when you're on a diet. That way, you know if you're making progress — and you reinforce your success by "seeing" it right away.

9. Strict adherence to a diet is necessary for success. If you can't resist a gargantuan dinner on a Saturday night and then going out for a hot fudge sundae the next night, you might as well forget about the whole thing.

Now, how many of those statements do you consider to be true? My guess is that most people who have been on diets would say that at least six or seven of them are true — and probably all of them. In the workshops I conducted, my guess proved correct.

The truth is that all of them are false.

Not only are they false, but if you believe in the truth of even *one* of those statements, that belief in itself could well be responsible for the failure of all your previous dieting efforts.

That is no exaggeration, but a very conservatively stated fact, based on innumerable observations by myself and others. If, for instance, you said to yourself, "Yes, my problem is that I need to lose 25 pounds," then I say to you that that one belief has probably undermined and destroyed all your dieting efforts, without you ever being aware of why they ultimately failed and why you are overweight today.

If you said to yourself, "True," after reading as few as three or four of those statements, that tells me your mental set virtually *guaranteed* that all your previous dieting efforts would fail.

Yet, I would guess that these "Deadly Myths," as I call them, are implicit in about nine out of ten dieting books and that even many doctors would regard most of those statements as true. It's no surprise, then, that losing weight and keeping it off is so difficult.

Embarking on a journey to slenderness with your mind packed with those beliefs is equivalent to setting off on an Arctic exploration believing that the North Pole is a tropical rain forest: doomed to failure because you don't understand the territory.

The fundamental reason, then, why the Prevention System of Natural Weight Control is much more likely to succeed than any other reducing plan you have tried, is that *we're going to unload these failure-insuring myths from your mind.*

And as we do that, we are going to replace them, one at a time, with new insights into the reality of weight control. More important, *we're going to arm you with new tools and skills that have been specially designed for successfully coping with weight problems,* just as the gear of an Arctic explorer or a mountain climber is specially designed to cope with his special environment.

To put it another way, the secret of success of this new approach is that there is no diet to follow. Instead of trying to artificially and drastically change the kind and amount of food you're accustomed to eating — an attempt which both of us know is doomed to failure — we are instead going to change *you.*

I don't mean we're going to try to psychoanalyze you or guru-ize you or change your personality. It's nothing as complicated or as ambitious as that.

What's going to happen as you read this book is that you'll learn some stark truths about weight control that are so obvious — and so important — you'll wonder why so few people seem to be aware of them.

You'll learn how to discover the "hidden" habits that have been defeating all your efforts to control your weight. You'll learn how to change those habits quickly and without using willpower. Intelligence, yes; imagination, yes; perseverance, absolutely — willpower, no.

You'll learn how to make these changes of habit much easier by applying a simple and perfectly safe technique of self-hypnosis.

You'll learn how to get more exercise than you ever dreamed possible — and without straining yourself.

You'll learn how to stop being obsessed by food and intimated by your appetite.

These insights and skills that you'll learn will prove to be more effective in helping you reach your goals than any "diet" yet devised. Soon, you'll probably be chuckling to yourself when friend after friend asks you what diet you've been following to lose all that weight.

They'll just never understand when you say, "I have no diet."

2

A Blueprint, Tools, and Skills

If you are like most of the people who read and used this book when it was still in the manuscript stage, you probably think it's mighty strange that the statement "My problem is that I need to lose weight" is considered false.

If you get nothing else from this book, you must appreciate the utter falsity — and the hidden trap — in that statement.

And why is it false?

Because, dear reader, if you are like me and 99 out of 100 people who are over 30 and overweight, you have *already* lost weight. It's a safe bet that you have dieted strenuously at least 3 or 4 times and maybe 30 or 40 times. And during at least one of those assaults on your waistline you probably came very close to reaching your ideal weight. At least, I'd venture, you managed to shed a good 15 pounds or so.

And then what happened?

See what I mean?

If your problem was *truly* that you needed to lose weight, your problem would have been solved a long time ago. It may, in fact, have been solved five times over!

But it would have been *really* solved only if you needed to lose weight in the sense that an unemployed person needs a job. When he or she gets the job, the problem ceases to exist.

Now, suppose for a minute that a good friend of yours is in

fact unemployed and asks you if you can get him a job with your company. But suppose you also know that person has been fired from three jobs in the last four years. If you are a true friend, it would not be at all helpful of you — in fact, it would be detrimental to your friend's future — to agree with him that his problem was that he needed a job. What's wrong is that he can't *keep* a job. So his real problem, *the one that needs to be worked on,* is not getting a job, but changing the pattern of behavior that is repeatedly undermining all his attempts to get a career going.

It's the same for you and me and everyone else who can't keep their weight where it belongs. The problem is not our waistlines, but our behavior.

If you are not yet convinced, imagine for a minute that I could give you a magical incantation right now that would cause 15 pounds to suddenly vanish from your body. Now stand back from your ego for a minute and look at yourself and your track record of weight control over the years and ask yourself: what are the honest-to-goodness odds that this individual you see is going to keep that weight off for more than a few months?

Would you be willing to bet even money that within six months he or she will have gained back at least 5 to 10 pounds, and from 10 to 15 pounds within a year?

Going by all the statistics I've seen coming out of studies of dieters, you couldn't go wrong with a bet like that.

Because having lost their weight, at least four out of five dieters immediately revert to the same behavior that got them fat in the first place. And the sad fact is that no matter how many times they go through this cycle, *most dieters never realize that they are guaranteeing their ultimate failure by attacking their bellies instead of their behavior.*

The idea of changing your behavior may sound difficult or even a little scary. But it isn't. The particular behavior patterns we'll be going after are only those which impinge directly on your weight. For the most part, changing these behavior patterns involves nothing more than modifying certain habits you have — often, habits you don't even know you have. Most people have never even thought twice about these habits — perhaps not even once, because a number of them are performed almost unconsciously.

But how does one go about changing habits, anyway? Especially when you may not even be aware that you have them? The answer is through the use of those *tools* and *skills* we mentioned before.

Probably right about now you are wondering — and justifiably — "How difficult is it going to be for me to change my habits, to lose weight and keep it off? Tools or diets — I don't really care which I use — but I want it to *work*! The thing is, I'm not that great in the willpower department. So how hard is all this going to be for a person like me?"

The honest answer to that question is: *surprisingly easy.* But those words need a little explanation.

Making a hard job easy. Let's say, by way of illustration, that you have decided to do a major remodeling project in your home. And you're going to do it entirely on your own. Doing the job you have in mind will require you to cut, sand, finish, and install wood; install a new tile floor; install exterior siding; install insulation; install a suspended ceiling; and finally, do a lot of staining and painting.

Now, does that sound difficult? I don't know about you, but it does to me, because I never learned how to do that kind of work with any proficiency at all, or even without proficiency.

To a carpenter, on the other hand, a job like that is ridiculously easy.

You're not a carpenter, you say? Fine. But let's suppose for a minute that you enrolled in a carpentry class that met twice a week for a whole year. And as the months passed, you developed not only a knowledge of the principles of carpentry, but actual experience in following a blueprint and working with wood and other materials, logging quite a few hours of hands-on experience in many phases of remodeling and building. And suppose that at the conclusion of the year, you went out and bought a set of first-rate tools and some proven plans that you could follow in doing your remodeling project.

At *that* point, you still wouldn't be a full-fledged carpenter, but you *would* be possessed of the skills and tools (and the confidence to go with them) that you'd need to make your project a success. And in *that* sense, the job that seemed almost impossible a year ago has now become, in a manner of speaking, easy.

That's just a long-winded way of saying that when you have the right blueprints, tools, and skills, any job that is not extraordinarily complicated can be successfully carried out in a very methodical way.

Most of us would regard our bodies as being at least as important as our houses. Yet, when it comes to remodeling *them,* we usually go about the project as if it were some silly game, instead of a major project whose success could bring us enormous gratification and heightened enjoyment of living.

We attack the job with no skills or tools whatsoever. And the only blueprint we have — in most cases — is a greased-lightning miracle diet published in a magazine or maybe one of those endless diet books written by doctors who couldn't get an article published in a medical journal if their lives depended on it.

The result, we all know from experience, is the same we'd get if we tried to build a new porch out of a pile of odd scraps of lumber, a box of assorted nails and screws left over from a garage sale, and a roll of adhesive tape.

Sure, you could get the porch to go up, but the first 10-mile-an-hour wind would bring the whole mess down.

And that's the way it goes with so many of our diet plans. Although everyone has enough common sense to realize that you can't build anything lasting without using the right materials and right tools, we often think that we can build ourselves new bodies in just that manner.

Oh, we *do* have one tool that we count on in our endless dieting, and we use it until it snaps under the strain — *willpower.*

Using willpower as your chief tool in dieting is like trying to drive nails into wood with your bare fists.

Combined with other qualities and assets — most of them new habits — willpower may have a place in the scheme of things after all. But to rely on it exclusively is probably the greatest mistake that any weight-reducer could ever make.

Now that we've come to grips with yet another of the "Deadly Myths" of dieting, let me add that the concept of willpower *in general* is highly overrated. I know that no one ever wrote a poem or built a sailboat or closed a big sale or raised three children on the strength of willpower. Desire, perseverance, patience, and the right skills are the kind of assets that get important things done. That goes for losing weight, too.

As a final note on this theme — before we begin to actually give you the blueprints, tools, and skills you'll need to be a successful reducer — you really ought to ask yourself how important it is to your future happiness to slenderize and stay that way. Does it have a really high priority among your other goals?

Given an either-or choice, would you rather be fat and drive a Cadillac or be slender in a Chevy? Would you rather have a big diamond ring around your chubby finger — or a simple gold band around a slender finger? Would you rather live in a house that was 50 percent bigger than your present house — or have a belly that was 10 percent smaller than the one you currently have?

These questions require serious answers, because if losing weight is not a real priority item with you, you might as well give the whole idea up right now. Because *anything* that you do in life, that you are going to do well, requires a certain amount of honest preparation and work. Whether it is skiing or driving a car or selling real estate or raising children, if you're going to make a good job of it, you have to bring something to the task besides the initial impulse to do it. Other people can give you advice and boost your confidence, but only *you* can provide the motivation.

Are you ready to put in some real work? I hope so. After all, aside from the enormous pleasure that being slender gives us, it is generally agreed that maintaining the right weight is of major importance in avoiding such common degenerative conditions as heart disease, high blood pressure, maturity-onset diabetes, low back pain, foot pain, gout, and even arthritis.

Isn't it worth a little time and effort, then, to achieve all those health benefits — and to *look* better besides?

3

Why Am I Eating This?

Did you ever wonder *why* you eat too much?

Most people to whom I ask this question reply with an answer something like one of the below:

"My appetite is too big."

"I'm a glutton, I suppose."

"I guess I'm just hungry all the time!"

Would your answer be similar? Do you think that your hunger is some kind of mad, starving beast? Well, relax; it isn't.

What if I told you that a very substantial amount of your eating is done without any sense of hunger whatsoever?

What effect would it have on your attitude toward your eating problem to know that it is perfectly possible for you to eat substantially less than you do now and never once get into a brawl with a hungry stomach? . . . Would it make you feel *good?*

All of us are familiar with some instances where we eat even though we're not particularly hungry. Sometimes we may be absolutely stuffed, but we still go on eating. Usually, we think of this happening when we are enjoying a very special meal at a fine restaurant in the company of good friends, or a Thanksgiving dinner. That kind of once-in-a-while indulgence is nothing to worry about. But few of us seem to realize that *eating when we're not really hungry is something we do almost every single day of our lives.* Eating without hunger is so commonplace that we do it almost unconsciously, and for a very wide range of reasons.

If you want to lose weight, and keep it off, it is absolutely essential for you to become aware of when, where, and why you are eating without hunger. *Once we have identified this behavior, we have at the same time found ourselves a wonderful opportunity for reducing our intake of food without fighting our hunger or depriving ourselves of needed nourishment.* In the next chapter, we'll begin to arm you with the skills you need to change your behavior and take advantage of this opportunity, but before we do that, we must become aware of exactly what it is we are going to change.

One of the first things we did in our diet workshops was to ask all the participants to keep a daily log of what they ate. But the important thing was not the total amount of what they ate — since everyone's caloric needs are different — but when, where, and under what circumstances they ate.

We also asked each participant to write down exactly how they felt before, during, and after each instance of eating, whether it was a meal, a major snack, or simply a quick nibble of this or that.

Each reader would be well advised to do the same thing for himself, but experience tells me that precious few people are actually going to do that. So instead, we'll review the experiences of our workshop participants in the expectation that each reader will probably be able to spot his own behavior patterns reflected in those of the workshop participants.

Way out in front as the occasion for eating without hunger was snacking while watching TV, generally between the hours of half-past eight and eleven o'clock in the evening.

"As soon as the first or second commercial goes on for the movie of the night, I get an uncontrollable desire to raid the refrigerator," one woman said, and at least half the other participants nodded their heads vigorously.

"Do you feel hunger at that time?"

"No, not at all. It's only been about two hours since I've finished eating dinner." Again, many of the other participants nodded.

"In between programs," another woman said, "I get an uncontrollable urge to get a bowl of pretzels and potato chips, set them down in front of me, and munch away."

"Do you feel hunger at that time?"

"To tell you the truth, sometimes I can still feel my dinner digesting in my stomach, but that doesn't seem to matter."

In fact, all the participants admitted that before TV snacking, they definitely were not hungry in the sense that their stomachs were uncomfortable, let alone growling.

In my own case, when I examined when and why I was eating, I realized that the desire for food was not coming from my stomach at all, but from my head. Even more specifically, it often seemed to stem from my *mouth.* Somewhere between the hours of about eight and midnight, I would — sometimes more than once — get a kind of dissatisfaction or itchiness or uneasiness and — entirely without thinking about what was going on — I would habitually start flinging open pantry doors, gazing inside the refrigerator, and taking quick looks inside the freezer.

Further reflection revealed that after eating whatever I chose (which meant whatever was handy) I rarely felt satisfied in any meaningful way. Rather, I felt uncomfortable. Ironically, even though I would often be uncomfortable, I would also feel a desire to eat still *more* food. Why, I'm not exactly sure, except that my digestive processes apparently swung into action after tasting the snack and protested being trifled with.

Many workshop participants said they typically nibbled on food while they were preparing dinner. It wasn't that they were really hungry or that they couldn't wait to sit down for the meal, but just having their fingers in all that food made it seem somehow logical to slip a few mouthfuls of this and that down the hatch.

In fact, whether cooking or not, a surprising amount of eating without hunger proved to be taking place either at the kitchen counter or right in front of an open refrigerator. Clearly, the mere proximity of food is motive enough to put it into your mouth, just as if the tonsils were a powerful magnet and the food, iron filings. Honest-to-goodness hunger has nothing to do with it.

Several participants said they ate when they were not hungry because their spouses were eating (whether *they* were actually hungry or not is another story), and they felt that it was unfriendly or uncooperative to refuse to share a snack with them. The temptation to do this is especially strong among people who may not spend a great deal of time with their spouses. Since all our workshop participants — the overwhelming number of whom were women — worked every day, these little moments of sharing probably had a special value. Still, the bottom line is that *they were eating when they were not hungry.*

One of the most common causes of eating without hunger — real, physical hunger — is loneliness or depression. There is something about the act of eating which is a kind of balm for these negative feelings, albeit a very transitory balm. What's more, what a person conditioned by habit to eat without hunger chooses at these moments is almost never healthful food. Almost invariably, it is cake, pie, ice cream, or chocolate — something *sweet.* Which means, of course, very high in calories.

Eating triggered by loneliness can be a powerful reflex, but *everyone* feels lonely or depressed from time to time, yet not everyone eats in response to these negative emotions. It follows that reflexive eating without hunger in response to these emotions is a *learned* behavior, not an instinctive behavior, and can therefore be *unlearned.* Even better, because eating does nothing in the long run to solve loneliness or depression, that kind of behavior can be replaced by more positive actions which enhance your ego as they diminish your hips.

Many workshop participants reported that after keeping a diary for a few days, they realized a major cause of eating without hunger was simply boredom. Eating, besides everything else you can say about it, is, after all, something to do. And food processors use every trick in the book to give food amusement value. They make snacks very crunchy, very salty, and then imbue them with exotic artificial flavors and colors. Soda pop and other beverages have a high amusement value. Popcorn, while certainly not a junk food, can nevertheless be abused when it is eaten not as a snack when you are hungry, but simply because you are bored and feel that your teeth and tongue need something to play with.

Ritualistic overeating at special occasions seems to be natural and is nothing to worry about, really. But many of us have a way of promoting every possible event to "special occasion" status. At one company where I worked, it was traditional for members of the office staff to bring in cakes on the occasion of someone's birthday. Somehow, these treats were always super-rich productions like Dutch chocolate cakes. If there was no cake, there was bound to be something like custard-filled doughnuts. That meant that about a dozen times a year, most of the office staff was indulging in three or four hundred calories — even though they weren't the least bit hungry, as these cakes were generally served at about ten in the morning. Eventually, the custom stopped, apparently for two reasons. First, many people became concerned about this pointless eating without hunger and second, a number of office workers were getting headaches or attacks of reactive low blood sugar in the wake of eating rich cakes and pastries in the morning.

Another version of this same general phenomenon often occurs when people visit each other's homes, not for major occasions, but simply for a brief social visit. At these times, it is often considered mandatory for the hostess or host to serve up vast quantities of food, nearly always including pastries and cakes. More likely than not, the people indulging in this food are not really hungry, and would be content with a cup of coffee, but the combination of social ritual and the sheer physical presence of heaps of food piled in front of them triggers yet another instance of eating without hunger.

You don't necessarily have to be at someone's house or a restaurant to find yourself being cued into irrational eating patterns. It could happen just a few steps from where you're sitting right now. Many people find it almost impossible to walk past the refrigerator without opening it and looking inside to see if anything catches their fancy. Hunger, of course, has nothing to do with it; the mere sight of the refrigerator door triggers the conditioned response of opening it. Three out of four times, probably, the door is closed without anything having been eaten, but the person who does this six or eight times a day is probably going to grab something and eat it at least once or twice.

In the next few chapters, I'm going to teach you how to avoid eating without hunger. At least I'm going to try. But before I do that, I'd like you to answer the following questions:

1. Did any of the instances of eating without hunger sound familiar to you?
2. Did any of those instances seem *very* familiar?
3. If you had a minute to think about it, could you come up with at least one personal example of eating without hunger I *didn't* mention? (Like eating the kids' left-overs . . . eating the potato chips that unexpectedly came with the hamburger you ordered . . . eating pop-corn at the movies?)
4. Does it seem to you that eating is too important to your health and well-being to be carried out in a semicon-scious state?

If you answered *yes* to all of the above questions, you are now ready to learn how to change your behavior.

4

If You Really Want It, You Can Have It

Remember the old saw about counting to ten before saying anything in anger?

The idea behind that musty adage is that most impulses to swear or yell at someone are so fleeting that if you simply think about something else for a little while, they will evaporate. And why bring down the wrath of the Almighty or lose a friend because of a fleeting impulse?

Nowadays, swearing isn't considered terribly sinful, while speaking out sharply is often said to be downright therapeutic. But when it comes to *eating* on impulse, no change in social customs can excuse the calories consumed.

And what this short but important chapter is going to do is simply teach you a fancy way of counting to ten before you give in to a fleeting impulse to push something into your mouth.

Let's say you're cruising by the refrigerator and lo and behold the door flings itself open. My, isn't that cup of custard interesting? *Very* interesting. And you know what? I'm hungry! I mean, really. After all, didn't I skip breakfast . . . day before yesterday? . . . Ooo, but I'm supposed to be losing weight. . . . But I'm hungry, dammit! I can eat when I'm *hungry,* can't I?

When you get into a situation like that, you're in trouble. Because one thing most people can't stand is to feel *deprived.* And no matter how fleeting the eating impulse may be, it usually gets its way by mounting a horse called "I really deserve this!" Here's what to do when you are confronted with that classic situation:

Tell yourself that if you are *really* hungry, you can certainly eat. All you have to do is wait seven minutes. Close the refrigerator door, knowing that the food is still going to be there seven minutes later, and then go do something else. Open a magazine, listen to some music, do anything you want to, as long as it gets you out of the kitchen or whatever room the confrontation occurs in.

Seven minutes later, if you still want that food, go and eat it. Maybe you really *are* hungry. Maybe not, but eating at that point may well be better for your reducing program than feeling deprived.

That delaying tactic, or balk, as baseball fans might like to call it, is one of the standard techniques taught by many behavioral psychologists treating people with eating problems. Different practitioners recommend different waiting times, but I have chosen seven minutes because if the delay is a round figure like ten minutes, there is a tendency to regard it as a concept rather than ten actual minutes. "I'll just wait a little while and then go eat it." If you think like that, "a little while" is liable to turn out to be 30 seconds. In practice, I've found that seven minutes is usually time enough to do the job, yet not so long as to be intimidating.

But even more important than really waiting seven minutes is to understand that the idea of this delay is not to somehow "trick" you out of your desired food. All you're doing is *testing* your impulse to see if it's sincere. If it is, act on it with an easy conscience. You haven't lost at any game. Whether you eat it or not, you've won, because you've done it *your way.*

One woman said this technique was the same idea parents try to get across to their teenage daughters when they are the recipients of sweaty propositions. "It's a question of self-respect. If we want our children to respect their bodies," the workshop participant said, "we should respect *our* bodies, too." I like that.

Winning without willpower. Let's now take a slow-motion look at the "showdown" at the refrigerator, to better understand what's really happening, and come up with some special moves we can utilize in executing the seven-minute delay technique.

There you were, walking through the kitchen, and the next thing you knew, you had opened the refrigerator door. Were you *hungry* when you opened the refrigerator? Hungry, shmungry, just about every time you pass that refrigerator you open it, don't you? And *why?* The answer is easy: it's a *habit!*

Right now I want you to get an image of yourself opening the refrigerator door and looking inside. As you see yourself in your mind's eye, realize that what you are doing is an unconscious — or at best, semiconscious — habit. You are acting like a laboratory mouse that spends half its waking hours making meaningless gestures like pressing a lever because it has been conditioned to do so. Now see an image of yourself as a giant laboratory mouse standing on its hind legs looking into your refrigerator, twitching its nose like crazy and reaching out for food because a graduate student in psychology has taught it to do so whether it is hungry or not. . . . *How do you like being a mouse?*

Actually, it's no great disgrace to do something out of habit. We do it all the time, when we nod at people, smile, straighten a stack of papers, or begin singing as soon as we step into the shower.

The difference between doing those things and opening the refrigerator door and snatching food is that smiling at people and singing in the shower aren't harmful. In fact, they're probably *good* habits. Most important, singing in the shower never increased the size of anyone's rear end the way grabbing food from the refrigerator does.

Picture yourself as a giant mouse again, nose quivering, eyes all beady, standing in front of the refrigerator. Picture it vividly . . . then let it slowly dissolve from your consciousness.

Suddenly it's *you* standing in front of the refrigerator. Intelligent, hard-working you. The apex of evolution. Made in God's image. Anyway you look at it, that's a mighty big brain you've got tucked inside your skull. A creature quite like you came up with the theory of relativity. Discovered the atom, wrote *Don Quixote,* and figured out how to eradicate smallpox from the face of the earth. There you are, in all your majestic humanity, standing in front of the refrigerator eyeballing a cup of custard.

Somewhere in your brain is the knowledge that losing the blubber on your body is one of the most important things you can do to enjoy a happier future. The day your weight begins to go down, in fact, every moment of your life will be happier. Every day you become healthier. Every day you will increase your energy and endurance. Every day you will become more attractive to yourself and to your friends. . . . But the part of the brain that knows this is not the only part of your nervous system that's working. In fact, the habit part, the semiconscious part, is red-hot. The mouse part of you. The part that does things without thinking, the part that keeps you eating when you don't want to eat.

It's very undignified, really. Who wants to fight a mouse? So do what any self-respecting *Homo sapiens* would do: simply walk away, instantly causing that mouse to disappear. It's not a willpower struggle, really, because as you leave the scene, you make a mental note that you will renegotiate the entire matter in precisely seven minutes. (Unless, of course, you are then otherwise engaged. I mean, why go out of your way to keep an appointment with a mouse?)

Clop. The refrigerator door just closed.

Klack. The door of the kitchen cabinet is shut.

Clong. That was the top of the cookie jar.

Now what? Without any further ado, not even a little dab of ado, haul your bones out of the kitchen.

What you do next depends on your individual interests. Do you love music? Get out your favorite record, slip it on the hi-fi, and listen to a couple of songs. But do it with a little finesse. If your favorite tune is the fourth cut on side A, put the needle at the beginning of the record. Now, if after seven minutes you want to take the record off before it gets to the part you like most, fine. That's part of the bargain. Like I said, you won't be losing, or suffering any kind of defeat. But maybe, just maybe, you'll find yourself wanting to hear your favorite part of the record a little more than you want that custard. In fact, there's a possibility that after five minutes or so, you'll have forgotten about that custard completely. You may not even think about it again until you go to bed, when the whole incident will bring a very self-satisfied smirk to your face.

Like to read? Find a new magazine or book, take it into the living room or bedroom, and plunge right in. Have you noticed that lately you haven't been able to find time to do the reading you really want to do? Well, you've just found that time.

Or maybe there's something in the workshop or in the sewing basket that you've been wanting to do for a couple of weeks. Here's the chance you've been waiting for. A very special kind of time that is reserved for doing exactly and exclusively what you want to do most. Oil your gun. Hang a picture. Paint a picture. Sit on your husband's lap. Teach your dog a new trick. Carry out the trash. Do the laundry. The ironing. Call your sister. See how many sit-ups you can do. Take the dog for a walk. Write a letter to your son. A letter to the editor. Vacuum the rugs. Get out the Sears catalog and decide what clothing you're going to buy when you lose your first ten pounds.

My brother Barry, a psychotherapist, advises people who want to lose weight to find a new hobby and really get involved in it. You can see why. If you have nothing to turn to except your TV, you're going to be in trouble. Because TV doesn't involve you the way real activities do. The first time a commercial break flashes on the screen, you're apt to say "Time's up!" and run back to the refrigerator or the cookie jar.

The activity you choose may be something you've been pursuing casually for quite a while. In the back of your mind, you've had the idea that it would really be fun to go at this hobby flat out, and if that's the case, now's the time to stomp on the accelerator. Buy the latest books about it. Go shopping for new equipment. Join a club. Tackle a really challenging but satisfying project.

You see, having a hobby is worth a lot more to you as a person with an eating problem than merely filling in seven minutes' time. In my own case, the hobby or interest that I took up when I went on a weight-reducing program was jogging. Now of course, any kind of exercise hobby is going to be doubly valuable, because it burns up calories while it keeps your mind busy. But when I got into jogging, I got into it *mentally* as well as physically. When I wasn't running, I was often thinking about it. I would read *Runner's World*, not just once, but two or three times. I even daydreamed about running. In short, as my brother Barry put it, I was "obsessed" with it. And he thought this was important because people who are trying to reduce often become obsessed with *food* — if they weren't before. And if you walk around all day thinking about food, you're going to be excruciatingly vulnerable to its charms, real or imagined. You're much better off daydreaming about swimming or quilting or building the addition on your home or having your sheep dog win Best in Show or learning to develop and print your own film.

One of the best obsessions to become a prisoner of is gardening. I would recommend it emphatically for anyone who has an eating problem during the day. Gardening not only gets you out of the kitchen, it gets you out of the house. It gives you exercise and perhaps most important of all, it gets your hands dirty. Hobbies that keep your hands busy, dirty, greasy, or wet, and therefore unable to reach into the refrigerator, are the best hobbies of all. During the evening, you can lavish loving attention on your pet, your indoor plants, your sculpturing or oil painting.

The best part about this whole approach is that you've used a no-win confrontation between food and willpower as a springboard to launch you into activities that will not only help you lose weight, but will add a lot of enjoyment to your life and make you feel much better about yourself.

5

Make It Easy on Yourself

No matter what kind of work we hope to do, we can make it easier on ourselves if we get organized first.

If it's tools we're going to need, we get them together and put them within easy reach. If the work we are going to do involves moving from place to place, we remove everything blocking efficient movement — first. Imagine, for a moment, what it would be like to try to do a household job with your tools scattered all over the house, the garage, and the yard. Or imagine trying to play tennis with beer cans and newspapers scattered all over the court.

If *those* examples seem silly, imagine how silly it is to try to do something as important as losing a substantial amount of weight without first getting yourself organized. Yet, that is exactly what most of us (including myself) have done in the past, with the predictable result of stumbling over all sorts of impediments . . . and finally getting so angry and frustrated that we simply give up.

Think of your weight-loss program as a journey. There is a long road ahead of you. But fortunately, right now, you can decide whether or not that road is going to be full of potholes, bumps, debris, and unmarked turns, or if it is going to be a well-paved, well-lit, well-marked path to success.

Sure, if you try hard enough you can get there just the same, but which would you rather be, an engineer or a human bulldozer?

You already have at your disposal a lot of the information you'll need to engineer a smoother path to weight loss and permanent weight control. That information consists of a knowledge of your own eating habits. You've become aware of the fact that a lot of the eating you do is carried out in what I call a semiconscious state, and is not motivated by real hunger, but simply habit and shallow impulses. Then you learned how to change some of those habits and how to *test* those impulses to find out if they are legitimate or phony. What we are going to do in this chapter is learn how to make it *easier* to change those habits, and reduce the number of phony impulses we have to contend with.

Localize your eating. You have already thought about circumstances which lead you to eat, other than mealtime. Now I want you to think about *where* you eat, other than your dining room table. We asked the participants in our workshop to do this, and here are some of their answers:

"I do 90 percent of my snacking sitting on the sofa watching the television," Marie said. Many others nodded in agreement.

"Standing right in front of the refrigerator," Stan said. "It is amazing how much I can eat, just standing there. Sometimes I don't even close the door. I keep the door open with the elbow of the same arm I'm using to eat!"

"At the kitchen counter, usually when I'm preparing dinner."

"I like to eat in bed, and there is nothing I like better than to eat crackers with peanut butter while I'm reading."

"This may sound strange, but I like to eat most when I'm driving. I'll stop into a Seven-Eleven store and buy some cupcakes or maybe a whole box of cookies and eat them while I'm driving."

Some people eat more than they need to, and frequently more than they want to, when they're eating dinner. We will get to that challenge a little later, but by far the greatest amount of impulse eating occurs *between* meals, and is almost always done at places *other* than the table where meals are eaten.

You've already made a deal with yourself that if you are *really* hungry, you can have it. So what we are going to do now is give you a new way to further "legitimize" your eating. Make this new deal with yourself: if you have decided that you really want to eat something, and if you have waited seven minutes after your initial eating impulse, you may eat it *only* if you do so seated at your dining room table.

There is no deprivation of food involved here. Far from it. Instead, you are going to enjoy your food in proper fashion. Whatever it is you have decided to eat, put it on a plate, or in a bowl, take it to the dining room table, sit down, and thoroughly enjoy every mouthful.

I guarantee that doing this will not increase the caloric content of your snack one bit: gobbling your food in front of the refrigerator is every bit as fattening as eating it from Bavarian china set on Spanish linen on your French provincial table.

Why go to all that trouble? Precisely because it *is* trouble. Going through that routine forces you to become acutely conscious of what you are doing. If your desire for food is legitimate, and not merely part of some mindless habit pattern like eating crackers while you watch TV in bed, it will not seem like any great ordeal to set the table and eat as if you really mean it. But if you are only kidding yourself, it may well seem like more trouble than it is worth. And often, that is exactly what happens.

Remember, the idea behind this is not to deprive you of food that you really want, only to make sure that you really want it. Surely, if you really want it, spending a single minute serving your food in a normal way is not unreasonable. And when you eat, you may do so with an absolutely easy conscience, because in all likelihood, your desire for that food is legitimate: hunger, not habit.

When you eat . . . eat! Now that you have become more conscious about *where* you eat, consider this question: Do you ever engage in snacking or even full-scale eating while you are doing something else? Or, looking at it another way, do you do anything *else* while you are eating? If so, what?

"I play cards once a week, and I just love to snack while I play," Sally said.

"With me, it's watching TV, just like before," Marie said. "TV is more enjoyable when you are eating." "Sometimes the programs are so dumb!" Roberta added.

"I always eat popcorn when I go to the movies."

"I always have a couple of beers when I go bowling."

"I know it is bad manners, but I almost always read the newspaper while I'm eating dinner."

Do any of those responses sound familiar? Maybe you have your own special activities that seem to invite snacking. With me, as with some of the others, it was watching TV. Whether it was just a simple habit, or, like Roberta said, because the programs are usually so dumb, I can't say. Perhaps it was simply a habit left over from my childhood, when I used to eat dinner from a TV tray while watching cartoons or football games. In any event, there is no doubt that many of us employ eating as a kind of background music while we are doing something else, much as the smoker lights up when he gets into a heavy conversation or goes to a cocktail party.

So let's make another deal. If you are doing something other than sitting down to a meal, and you want to eat, you certainly can — but only if you stop what you're doing, go to the dining room table as before, and sit down and eat *while doing nothing other than eating.* If you're *really* hungry, you'll do it. If not, you won't. You'll prefer to keep on playing cards or watching the football game or reading your book.

As a kind of corollary to this principle, I must advise strongly against reading at the table. The more conscious you are of eating, the better off you will be. Your food will be much more satisfying when you are paying attention to it, looking at it, smelling it, feeling it, tasting it, chewing it, thinking about it.

When do you lose control? This next little bit of domestic engineering is related to those above, but asks the specific question: at what point in your daily schedule, or what time of the day, do you seem to do the most snacking? More than likely, it's the evening. Perhaps it occurs when you are watching TV, as we mentioned before, but right now I want you to think about the problem in a slightly broader perspective. In other words, it might be more effective to look upon a certain part of the day as your vulnerable *time,* rather than a vulnerable activity or place. Now, if you are in fact doing most of your snacking in the evening, say between the hours of nine and eleven, why not plan on *scheduling* some new kind of activity during those hours, something to reduce the total number of phony eating impulses you have to contend with? You could, for instance, schedule several evening trips to the Y every week, sign up for classes or clubs that meet at night, take up a new hobby or rekindle your interest in an old one that can take you away from all the familiar cues, like watching TV, that habitually spark those snacking impulses.

With me, the vulnerable time was between the hours of eleven at night and one in the morning. Usually, at that time, I'd be through my evening reading and writing and would watch TV until I couldn't keep my eyes open anymore. It was amazing how many trips I used to make to the refrigerator. There was no legitimate reason for me to be that hungry, so I thought about exactly what it was that was causing me to do all that uncontrollable snacking.

The major reason, I concluded, was simply that when it's late at night, and I'm tired, the most rational part of my mind rapidly becomes drugged. I'm a sucker for any fleeting impulse. But there might have been another reason, I concluded, and that was that I was eating in a kind of perverted attempt to stay awake. By shoveling sweet things down my throat, my blood sugar would rise and give me a temporary energy boost. Then I asked myself: *why am I staying up so late in the first place?* Why is it so important to watch those old movies I have seen so many times, or see who the next celebrity is going to be on the "Johnny Carson Show," when all it's doing for me is making me incredibly tired and causing me to eat like a maniac? I didn't have any answer to that.

Finally I got the idea of simply cutting those late hours out of my life, like hacking off a rotten limb from a tree, and replacing them with a couple of other hours during which I would be fresh, totally in control of my impulses, and not in the least inclined to snack. In other words, I started going to bed at eleven and waking up at half-past six, instead of going to bed at one and waking up at eight.

And that was one of the smartest things I ever did.

I was able to avoid a lot of impulse eating without getting into a "confrontation" with the food; I felt much more rested in the morning; and I found the new time I had created for myself in the morning to be ideal for jogging or writing, which I did on alternate days.

Out of sight, maybe out of mind. Have you ever found yourself eating something simply because it was *there?* I mean *right* there — smack under your nose. I guess we all have. Many of us impulse eaters are something like frogs, programmed by evolution to flick out their tongues whenever anything small enough to be slurped down moves into range of vision.

Why make it difficult on yourself by permitting all sorts of unwanted foods to entice you? If you really *want* food, you know where to get it. The idea is to keep it from *harassing* you.

What I suggest, therefore, is that you spend ten minutes or so doing a little redecorating and moving. Are there bowls of chips or pretzels or candies scattered around your house? Maybe they *do* add an interesting note of warmth or color to the decor, but imagine what they're going to do for the decor of your belly and hips. Get rid of them. Wrap them up and put them away. That even goes for bowls of fruit. Fruit is a good food, but no food, no matter how nourishing, should be eaten on the merest of impulses, simply because it is *there.*

What about your kitchen counter? Are there boxes of crackers, cookies? Packages of doughnuts? English muffins? Sweetened cereal? Perhaps a bottle of wine? Take a good, hard look.

I want you to put all those things away, but not just anyplace. Take all of them and put them in one special cabinet or drawer which will be, in effect, a fat-food compound. Preferably, this should be a cabinet that's a little bit out of your way or hard to reach. You won't be opening it by accident. And by having all those snacks in one place, instead of merely hiding them in the back of your regular cabinets, you won't be "accidentally" stumbling across a bag of pretzels while you're hunting for a can of tomato sauce.

But what about the kids, some people ask. They have to be able to get these snacks easily, don't they? To which I answer: *why?* Do they really *need* potato chips, pretzels, candy, and all those other empty-calorie foods? Maybe *they* think they do, but you know better. I'm not saying they can *never* have any pretzels or chips, only that they, too, should be conscious of what they are putting into their mouths. And it seems to me that if your children are so small that they can't reach food placed in a cabinet, then they ought to be *asking* you if they may have a snack in the first place.

As for the refrigerator, it would be nice if we could all afford two refrigerators, but lacking that, we can at least keep things arranged so that the high-calorie impulse items are consistently placed way in the back. Let's face it, even if you are abiding by your agreement not to grab anything out of the refrigerator until you've waited seven minutes, you're going to be making it that much easier on yourself if, when you *do* have to open the refrigerator for a legitimate reason, the first thing you see isn't a half-eaten blueberry pie ringed by bottles of Coca-Cola. The front of your refrigerator should be loaded with fruits, vegetables, and meat-and-potato-type leftovers. Likewise, the storage shelves on the inside of your refrigerator door should be restricted to carrying nonsnack items like eggs and butter. In the freezer compartment, put any ice cream or similar snacks behind the frozen meats and vegetables.

Signs of the new times. Now that you have done some engineering to make the road to permanent slenderness a little smoother, give some attention to helpful road signs. These road signs — you may be using anywhere from one to half a dozen — will be placed throughout your home, in places where there are critical "turns." I know it sounds a little corny, but many people find that domestic signs prove every bit as useful in preventing needless wrong turns as the road signs on a busy freeway. In fact, that's a good analogy, because just as a highway sign sort of jogs you out of the semihypnotic state that you sometimes fall into when zooming down the road mile after mile, a domestic sign can suddenly restore you to full consciousness as you drive down the road of daily routine.

WAIT SEVEN MINUTES. THANK YOU!

That was the sign one workshop participant placed on her refrigerator door. She reported it cut down the number of times she opened the door by about 25 percent. A man put a sign on his refrigerator door that read:

ARE YOU HONESTLY HUNGRY? FIND OUT

The sign I put in my own kitchen, taped to a cabinet, and written in large, colorful letters, was:

EAT IT AT THE TABLE, PLEASE

Notice that I'm not suggesting you put up signs saying things like "Don't eat it!" or "Do you want to stay fat?" For one thing, I don't believe much in negativity, or in threats, either. It's hard enough putting up with the negativity and harassment of others, so why should we have to insult *ourselves?* Be intelligent, polite; show respect for yourself.

I suggested to one woman who was having a difficult time getting into the habit of walking, that, among other things, she put a sign on her coat-closet door reading:

WANT TO LOSE SOME WEIGHT, RIGHT NOW?

But the sign she actually *did* put up read:

WEIGHT-LOSS EQUIPMENT ROOM

Use your imagination to decide what kind of signs you're going to use. In fact, spending a few moments at this will give you the added benefit of raising your consciousness of those places in your home where you're especially vulnerable. If you feel, for example, that you might "accidentally" fling open the cabinet door where you've stashed away snacks, label it with a sign reading simply:

FAT-FOOD COMPOUND

Or:

DRINK SOME WATER!

Or maybe just:

THINK!

One sign that sounds a little simplistic but really isn't is:

THINK THIN!

What that sign means is just what it says. Think that you *are* thin. Picture yourself as a slender person, an active person, a person with a perfectly normal appetite. It's a little bit like the hypnotic technique of imagining, for instance, that the pain *is* gone, which seems to be more effective than imagining that it's beginning to go away. Along these lines, I like the signs that Linda put up, the first on the inside of her front door, the second in her bedroom:

HOME OF THE WORLD'S CHAMPION WALKER

EVERY DAY I AM A NEW PERSON

Help your family help you. An absolutely incredible amount of eating without hunger is done for the simple reason that someone else in the family offers you food. I don't mean when they serve you a meal, but when they invite you to eat more than *you've* decided to eat, or at a time when you aren't particularly interested in eating. At the table, many of us say to our spouses or children things like:

"Want some more spaghetti?"

"Don't you like my muffins? They're delicious!"

"Finish your potatoes, Billy."

"Want to split that last piece of pie with me?"

"Is that all you're going to eat?"

If people are really hungry, if they really need more food, they don't have to be cajoled or even invited to eat it. When you invite them to do more eating, you are interfering with the functioning of their natural appetite control system, which is the most fundamental mistake that can be made.

But what if other people keep pushing food at *you?* Probably that's happening, and maybe more than you think. Wives do it, husbands do it, neighbors do it, hosts do it, and sometimes waitresses. The only people who *don't* do it are children, who have more common sense than we give them credit for. But if it's inappropriate for a child to encourage an adult to eat more, it's just as inappropriate — and perhaps even more inexcusable — for one adult to push food at another.

Therefore, what I suggest is that you simply ask other members of your household not to offer you food. Explain to them that you've decided to slim down and that the program you're following depends on not eating when you're not hungry. So to help you, would they please refrain from offering you second helpings, snacks, glasses of wine, even pieces of fruit.

At first, they will probably slip up. When they do, don't get angry. Just say, "No thanks, I don't want to eat when I'm not really hungry." That will gently remind them of what you told them before, without explicitly criticizing them. And you don't want to criticize anyone in your household at this time, because that will only increase the tension and make your new way of eating more difficult. The idea is to make it easy on yourself!

6

Wash Away Your False Hunger

By now, we all know that many of our impulses to eat are not triggered by true hunger, but by nonphysical factors ranging from a desire to be polite to a need to keep our hands busy. I'm sure many people realize that without having read this book.

But what most people do not realize is that a major reason for irrational eating behavior is the failure to recognize that *many impulses to eat something are misinterpretations of thirst — a desire, a real honest-to-goodness need, for water.*

Your body's need for H_2O is more urgent than its need for any other compound except O_2 — oxygen. Two or three days without water is enough to put anyone at death's door, while a single day without water can endanger the life of someone who is not in robust health. Intestinal infections causing diarrhea take the lives of more infants throughout the world than any other disease, but death is caused not by the bacteria per se, but by dehydration. It is entirely logical, then, that *nature has endowed us with an extraordinarily powerful thirst mechanism to insure that we get enough of this vital fluid.*

The big problem as far as our health and our waistlines are concerned is that *what we do when this thirst mechanism goes into operation is not what nature intended for us to do.*

I became aware of that shortly after I began the weight-control program described in this book. When I had an impulse to put something into my mouth when it wasn't time for a meal, I would wait for seven minutes or so and then observe what happened to the put-something-in-my-mouth impulse over that short stretch of time. But I did something else, too. Instead of just closing the refrigerator door and going down to my basement to listen to music, I would stand there for a while and try to analyze the exact nature of the impulse that had caused me to open the refrigerator door almost unconsciously.

When you're trying to analyze that kind of impulse, you may not have much success if you're too aggressive or direct in your analysis. So I did what I often do when confronted by a problem at work or in my personal life: I simply emptied my mind, slipping into a kind of instant meditation, but remaining sensitive to images, thoughts, or feelings that seemed to thrust themselves into my consciousness.

And when I did that, it dawned on me that the basic need which had taken me to the refrigerator was *dryness of my mouth and throat.*

What an amazing revelation that was! There I was, in the so-familiar posture: poised before the refrigerator door, my eyes wandering over the lighted contents, trying to decide what I felt like eating. What I *really* wanted — the desire that had brought me there — was not anything at all to be found in the refrigerator, but simply *water.*

But then — *why had I gone to the refrigerator?*

That was no great mystery, at least on one level of understanding. It was a conditioned response to a sensation of oral uneasiness which I had never before bothered to reflect upon. In other words, a stupid habit.

The eating-for-thirst syndrome. Closing the refrigerator door and analyzing my behavior further, I was quickly able to understand how I had fallen into that particular — and very fattening — habit. For one thing, eating food is more fun than drinking water. Besides swallowing something, you get to taste something, smell something, and chew something. And then, there are no ads on TV telling us that drinking water is an ecstatic experience. (Can you imagine an ad for "The Water Generation"?)

On a more physiological level, putting almost anything in your mouth and chewing it *temporarily* satisfies whatever uneasiness you may have in the space between your lips and stomach. It can even temporarily alleviate dryness, because saliva is generated in the process of mastication.

There's another reason, though, why we are able to habitually eat when our body wants us to drink and still not run into problems with dehydration. And that is that *many foods, including most of our favorite snacks, consist largely of water.*

A piece of apple pie, for instance, is by weight almost 48 percent water.
Cheddar cheese is 37 percent water.
Boston creme pie is 35 percent water.
Chocolate cake is 25 percent water.
Chocolate pudding is 65 percent water.
Potato salad, for all its calories, is 76 percent water.
Fruits such as cherries, apples, and peaches are between 80 and 90 percent water.
Even chicken and beef contain a lot of water — averaging about 60 percent.
Ice cream is 63 percent water.

After running the above through my head, I decided that the next time I found myself clutching the refrigerator door, I was going to shuffle over a few steps, turn on the faucet, and draw myself a big glass of cold water. Eureka! It was incredibly satisfying — even more so than sweet snacks, because water was what my body wanted and now I was giving it *the real thing!*

That discovery led to more understanding of how I had gotten in the habit of eating for thirst. Water, in our society, is something that enjoys the same status as a food that digging ditches does as an occupation. As a result, many people do not have a convenient supply of water they can enjoy drinking. No matter how crowded my own refrigerator was, one thing that was never in it was water. And there seemed to be something dull or even unappetizing about drawing water from the kitchen sink, which often contained stacks of dirty dishes.

For me, then, it became important first, to make sure that I had access to water that I could enjoy drinking, and second, to get into the habit of actually doing so.

I found that I could accomplish both these goals quite easily. I soon learned to disregard dishes in the sink and discovered that if I let the water run for about 15 seconds, my well would supply me with some very fine drinking material, entirely free of the off-odors I had always associated with water since the days when I had lived in Philadelphia. Meanwhile, I made it a point to fill up a glass with water and quaff the contents any time I was passing through the kitchen and began to feel even the remotest sensation of uneasiness in my mouth, throat, or stomach. Besides drinking a lot more plain water, I also began to drink one or two cups of coffee in the evening, which I had never done before. I found that coffee, probably because it is hot, has its own unique appetite-controlling effect. And since I have a very high tolerance for caffeine, no sleeping problem resulted.

The result of consuming a much greater quantity of water was that it became much, much easier for me to control my snacking behavior — particularly in the evening, which was the only time of the day when I really had a problem.

Each reader must figure out for himself how he is going to get good water and how he is going to get into the habit of drinking it. For many, this will prove to be remarkably easy. For others, it may mean buying a water filter or bottled spring water in order to get something that you can really enjoy drinking. It may also mean keeping a supply of clean, attractive drinking glasses handy at all times — perhaps right next to the refrigerator instead of in a cabinet. It might also mean taping a little sign to the refrigerator door that says:

HOW ABOUT
A NICE SLENDERIZING
GLASS OF WATER?

Now, it's possible that upon self-observation and experimentation, you will not be overly impressed with the idea that you're eating in response to a hidden craving for water. Just the same, our experience in weight-control workshops suggests that making it a point to drink a lot more water is one of the smart things to do in order to promote the success of your reducing program.

Ruth said that when she came home from work every day, she would be "ravenously hungry" and immediately go to the refrigerator and begin eating. When she very consciously poured herself a glass of water immediately upon arriving home, she found that it was remarkably effective in blunting or easing her hunger pangs — which turned out to be more like impulses than true hunger. It didn't abolish the problem, but it reduced the amount she ate by one-third to one-half.

Carol said that going to the water fountain frequently during the day and drinking small amounts of water in the evening made her stomach feel more satisfied with less food.

Based on many experiences, I have the impression that drinking more water is similar to getting more exercise, in the sense that the overall effect is to *normalize* your appetite. Exactly how it does this I'm not certain, but for many people, I *am* certain that it helps. Furthermore, the idea that water tends to normalize the appetite is entirely logical from the nutritional point of view, as it is likely that throughout most of our time on earth, we human beings were drinking a great deal more water than we are today. That was a result of much greater physical activity, which promotes thirst, and greater dietary dependence on greens, fruits, berries, vegetables, and sprouts, all of which have a very high water content.

What I urge you *not* to do is to try drinking four brimming glasses of water instead of eating your lunch or dinner. Like all the other crash programs that so many of us try, overdoing water will only backfire. Sometimes literally.

The trick of success here, in fact, is not to see how much water you can drink, but simply to drink the first few glasses. Once you do that, using very good water, you will see that it helps you, and you'll want to make it part of your daily routine.

7

Trash Your Fat!

I can see it now:

A skinny preschooler, slumped over a big wad of cold mashed potatoes. By this time, I had been playing with the potatoes so long it looked like a truck had run over them, but that didn't bother my mother a bit: "Eat those mashed potatoes! Don't you know there are children starving in Europe?"

That must have been a universal occurrence, because everyone in our diet workshop recalled a similar incident — although no one would admit playing the role of the mother in this scene!

We got a good chuckle out of that, but it wasn't so funny when I asked how many still found themselves eating just to clean their plates . . . and 11 out of 12 people raised their hands.

Eating food as an alternative to throwing it away is really a bizarre phenomenon, if you think about it.

First, as I asked the workshop participants: what do you think of the idea of using your mouth as a garbage disposal? I mean, really think about it for a minute and see how it feels.

Second, imagine the problem you face when you have a sudden and powerful impulse to put something into your mouth. Then, *consider what you're doing when you shovel food into your mouth when you don't feel so much as a fleeting impulse to eat, let alone real hunger.* You may even be stuffed, but there it is, that extra piece of meat, on your plate or Susan's or Bill's, and *something* takes control of your arm and the next thing you know the food is in your mouth.

The plate is clean. Goody. And you're fat.

But just acknowledging that plate-cleaning without hunger

occurs does not solve the problem, not by a long shot. Like any other habit, it needs to be worked on before it drops away. In this chapter, we're going to do that work.

As I was reviewing what I wanted to say in this chapter, I realized that I almost forgot to mention that, contrary to what your mother told you, cleaning off your plate (or someone else's) doesn't do the starving masses a lick of good. If anything, it's making their plight worse. Here's why: when you eat food you don't need and add fat to your body, you are raising the number of calories you will require daily to haul your body around. A person who is 50 pounds overweight requires about 700 more calories each day to pay the metabolic price of his poundage. So if you want to be strictly logical, cleaning up a plate is a good way to *starve* other people, not feed them.

Maybe so, you say, but isn't food *precious?* "There is something wrong with throwing food away," one person in our workshop said. "I know it may sound corny, but food is really the most valuable thing in the world and it seems like a crime to throw it away."

I can understand how someone can feel that way. Particularly if you were brought up during the depression or the war or if you were raised in the kind of family that practically worships food. But the truth is that although food may in fact be precious, although food may in fact be expensive, and although it does rub all of us the wrong way to see good food thrown out, *food is not scarce in the culture we live in.* Expensive, maybe, but not scarce.

Do you know what the biggest single problem facing the American farmer today is?

Too much food. At least according to my own analysis. Depending on weather conditions and export trends, certain crops from time to time may become relatively scarce, but the big picture is embarrassing overproduction, right across the board. Maybe "embarrassing" isn't the right word; as far as the small farmer is concerned, this overproduction is nothing less than ruinous. The supply of most staples is so great that the price the farmer receives is often barely enough to pay his out-of-pocket costs. As a result of the selective breeding of dairy cows, for instance, milk production per cow has risen to the point where only the most efficient operations are able to show a respectable profit. The net result is that thousands of dairy farmers are cashing out every year. Conditions would be a lot harder for farmers if the government didn't go to great lengths to keep excess food off the market. Many people don't realize it, but the government pays "diversion" money to many farmers not to raise crops on their land, restricts the amount which other farmers are permitted to grow, and then buys up large quantities of other foodstuffs in order to keep prices at a level where most farmers can survive. There is an orange grower in Southern California who gets fined thousands of dollars every year by the government for raising and marketing more oranges than his allotment calls for. Like I said, food may be expensive, but it isn't scarce.

As for those starving kids in Europe, they've all grown up now and belong to Weight Watchers. There are warehouses in Europe bulging at the seams with *thousands of tons* of powdered milk, butter, and other dairy products that no one wants to buy. Except the governments of Europe, which are committed like our own to keeping farmers in business even if they're producing more food than people can eat.

All this may strike you as being overdrawn, but I think it's important for all of us with eating problems to realize that it's no crime to throw away extra food. Sure, food is precious, but too much of anything can become harmful. There is no excuse, then, for eating food as an alternative to throwing it out. It's just a habit, a fattening habit.

We all do it. Right now I want you to stop and think of some situations where you typically sweep leftovers into your mouth. Stop reading and look up at the ceiling for a minute and try to think of three situations.

We asked that question in our workshops, and some of the answers we got were:

- "When my Bobby doesn't finish what's on his plate." And how often is that? "All the time!"
- "When I finish eating before my husband does, sometimes I'll sit there and keep picking, keep eating until he's done." And how often do you finish before he does? "All the time!"
- "If I'm eating potato chips out of a small bag, I may be satisfied with what I've eaten, but if there's only a few left, I eat them too. Why throw them away?"
- Ditto, with pretzels, cookies, nuts, etc.
- "If my husband pours me a beer, I'm usually filled after I drink half of it, but he says 'Go ahead and finish it' . . . and I do."

- "About once a month we go out to a restaurant and I like to order steak. It's always too much for me, but I force myself to finish it because it's so expensive."
- "When we go to Mario's for pizza, it's always too much, but it's so good I hate to see it go to waste, so I help finish it off."

Here are a few other examples of compulsive plate-cleaning in action:

- You open a package of three cupcakes, eat two, and feel satisfied. You eat the third because it's there.
- You're with friends in a restaurant and you've only eaten about half the food on your plate when you lose interest in it. But you go ahead and finish it because otherwise it will look as though you're sitting in front of a plateful of garbage.
- Everybody knows that strawberry shortcake kept in the refrigerator overnight dies a slow death and you only have one piece left so you put it out of its misery.

In some cases, the appropriate thing to do with leftovers is to immediately wrap them and put them away. In those instances, the best thing to do is to practically jump out of your seat, wrap the food or put it in a dish, and stow it.

But often, there isn't enough left to be worth storing or reheating. In most cases, the only sensible thing to do is to trash it.

But before we get to actually trashing our fat, we're going to do a very important exercise in food consciousness. I've done it myself and others have too, and although it may sound crazy, I assure you that it isn't. There is a real point to it. And it's fun besides.

Right now, I want you to get up, walk over to your refrigerator, and open it. Now reach inside, grab some food, and throw it in the trash. Go ahead, do it now. I'll wait. . . .

What did you throw out? A jar of olives that had only three or four left in the bottom? Half of a cheese sandwich three days old? Fine. How did it feel? I mean, were you nervous? Did you think you were wasting good money? Probably, you felt pretty good, like cleaning house a little. I'm doing this exercise along with you, by the way, and I got off pretty easy: a plastic tube full of hot Chinese mustard.

Now I want you to go back to your refrigerator, and this time choose *two* items and throw them *both* in the trash. Really do it. This is important. . . . Well, how did you make out? Was it painful? Or was it . . . in a strange way . . . kind of fun? Personally, I enjoyed it. I took half a can of V-8 juice that had been sitting in the refrigerator for a week and poured it down the drain, and threw the can in the trash with an old and almost-used-up bottle of low calorie salad dressing. Somehow, it feels good to get old food out of the refrigerator. It doesn't belong there.

Now for the conclusion of the exercise. Go *back* to the refrigerator. This time I want you to select something that has a lot of calories in it. Pick it up, bring it to eye level, take a good look at it and imagine what all those calories would look like on your cheeks, your belly, or your butt. Then say good-bye to the food . . . and *trash your fat!* Go ahead; you go to your refrigerator and I'll go to mine. I'll meet you back here in a minute.

Well, how did it feel? Terrific, right? "Liberating," was how Nick put it, describing how he had trashed three or four rich pastries that were left in a box a relative had brought over the previous day. "For the first time, I had a feeling that *I* was the master, not the food. . . . And it wasn't hard at all."

Just a minute ago, I had a liberating experience myself, specifically liberating a disgustingly sweet bottle of Japanese plum wine that had been sitting in my refrigerator for about a year. The funny thing is, although I *know* the techniques I'm describing here, just knowing them doesn't do you any good: you have to *practice* them. And I haven't practiced the food-liberating technique for quite a while now. Otherwise, I would have realized how stupid it is to keep a horrible-tasting bottle of wine in the refrigerator indefinitely just because you paid good money (all of $2.96) for it. And having done that, I noticed that there was a bottle of off-taste eggnog that had been sitting in the back of my refrigerator since someone gave it to me at a Christmas party. That went down the drain, too.

The point of that exercise was not really to get rid of food that you would otherwise eat. I would have never consumed that wine or eggnog anyway. And perhaps you chose to sacrifice a little bit of dried-out ice cream rammed into a corner of your freezer. No matter. The idea was simply to see what it feels like to throw food away, food that you don't really want. And to realize that it isn't all that difficult. And, perhaps, strangely satisfying.

The rest is easy.

Fat trashing in action. Now that you are fully conscious of the nature and extent of the plate-cleaning habit, and you realize that throwing away leftover food is neither sinful nor particularly difficult, you're in business. Let's say you're eating at home and the main course was spaghetti and meatballs. You've finished what was on your plate and feel quite satisfied. Not bloated, but satisfied. Little Timmy is still staring at at least half of what he started with, while your husband is finishing his second helping. In the middle of the table there is a serving dish that has one meatball in it and a little bit of spaghetti. "Go ahead and finish it off," your husband says with a mouthful of spaghetti. "It's just one meatball. And Timmy, you finish yours, too!"

Being fully prepared for this potentially fattening situation, you know exactly what to do. You immediately get up, fetch the one empty custard dish in your pantry, and fill it with the meatball and spaghetti that was on the serving plate. You put wrapping around it and put it in the refrigerator. "Why don't you go ahead and eat what's on Timmy's plate," your husband suggests. You wish you could put that away, too, but there's no more empty dishes. For a second, you feel like taking your husband's advice, because you went to all the trouble to make those delicious meatballs and Timmy doesn't appreciate them. Then you suddenly realize what it is you're contemplating: *making yourself fatter because there's no available storage dishes.* Is your *stomach* a kind of storage dish? You also realize that Timmy isn't exactly starving to death, and that he has in fact eaten all that his young, slender body really needs. Rather than being unappreciative, his stomach is smart enough to realize when it's had enough.

So you take away his dish and feed it to the dog. Or to the garbage can. Yes, meatball and all.

"Hey! What are you doing, throwing away a meatball?"

"Trashing my fat!"

Here's another domestic situation:

Your sister comes over to have lunch with you and your family and brings with her a large bag filled with hamburgers, milk shakes and french fries. The kids are wild about it and shout with glee. You're kind of underwhelmed with it but when your sister brings lunch over, what are you going to do?

One thing you can do is to remove the middle slice of bread from the Big Mac. Having read the chart at the back of this book, you know that a Big Mac has 540 calories, so by removing that piece of bread and some of the excess sauce from the burger, you're saving yourself about 100 calories, all of it from white bread, oil, and sugar. And now the fun starts.

"What are you doing?" your sister demands. "If I had known you weren't hungry, I would have gotten you a regular hamburger!"

"Well, I do have an appetite, but it will taste just as good without the extra bread."

Your sister gives you such a look.

Five minutes later, you've polished off the burger and about three-quarters of your vanilla milk shake. Your french fries (large-size bag) are about 50 percent intact. Noticing that the kids haven't finished their milk shakes either, you take yours and spill the remainder down the drain of your sink.

"*Now* what are you doing?" your sister wants to know.

'Oh, did you want the rest of the milk shake?"

"Of course not. I have my own."

"Well, I didn't want it, either."

"A fine example you're setting for the kids!" You chuckle, but inwardly. Very inwardly.

"Anybody want more french fries?" you ask. No takers.

You roll up the bag of fries and toss it half-way across the room into the trash. Two points.

"Are you trying to insult me?"

"No, sis, honest. I'm just trashing my fat!"

I've spelled these incidents out in some detail to emphasize the fact that when you begin trashing your fat, you're going to have more of a problem with other people than with yourself. Not having raised their food consciousness as you have, they are still in thrall of the clean-up-your-plate commandment. Handle their feelings with tact, in a very neutral way. Don't accuse them of trying to push food down your throat, even though you may sometimes feel that way. The way *they* see it, they're only being considerate.

Here is a scene at a restaurant:

Having had soup, a roll, a large salad, and a glass of wine, you are ready to run up the white flag by the time you're two-thirds of the way through your expensive veal dish. For a moment you think, gee, this is nice, tender veal, and the sauce is excellent. I really ought to finish it. Then, of course, you realize how *silly* that is. All you'll be doing is *ruining* a good meal by making yourself feel bloated. So you call it quits. The problem is, being in a restaurant, you can't remove what is left, and your waiter is nowhere in sight. And if that veal just keeps sitting in front of you, you have a feeling that you are going to attack it again.

What you do is take your knife and fork and lay them across your plate, in such a way that the handles become fully immersed in the sauce. Then you push your plate a few inches in front of you to signal to everyone that you're done eating, and finish off your glass of water.

Having done that, you feel quite relieved. And ten minutes later, it's not at all difficult for you to get up and leave the table with half a glass of wine still sitting in your glass.

"Aren't you going to finish that wine?"

"I've had all I really feel like drinking." In restaurants, it's *gauche* to talk about trashing your fat.

Here's a particularly tricky situation:

You had dinner at the home of some new friends, and later, the hostess serves coffee and homemade pound cake. She gives you a rather large piece, and when you're half-way through it, you realize that (*a*) the pound cake isn't really that good, and (*b*) you really don't want the rest of it. What are you going to do, leave half of it on your plate? It's practically like tacking up a sign that says "This pound cake leaves something, shall we say, to be desired."

Let's backtrack a little and see if it's possible to do a little engineering. For one thing, you could have asked for a very small piece, realizing that if the pound cake proved to be especially good, your hostess would ask you if you wanted more, and you could flatter her by saying "Yes, it's delicious!"

Now, in this particular case, she didn't ask you what size piece you wanted, so upon being handed the large slice, you could have said "Oh, I know I'll never be able to finish this!"

"Really? Are you still full from dinner?"

"Well, I just feel very *comfortable* right now, and lately my stomach seems to have shrunk."

So, if you decide not to finish it, no one is going to be surprised or insulted.

But let's assume that you didn't do either of these things and you're just sitting there looking at a couple of hundred calories worth of insipid cake. Or maybe it really *is* good, but you just don't feel like finishing it anyway. What you do in a situation like that is to quickly put up a "sign" of your own. "Mrs. Smith, I'm sorry that I have to waste part of your cake, but pound cake is so rich. It fills me up really fast."

Now you *could* say "Gee, Mrs. Smith, this pound cake is really *fabulous* but blah blah blah," but I wouldn't recommend that. If the cake is not really good, your hostess will almost certainly realize it and either think you're a liar or tell you so to your face: "You don't have to make excuses, this is a lousy recipe."

My advice is to be tactful, but honest, too. That is a good combination in many situations.

8

Mealtime: Plan, Don't Plunder

How many times have you gotten up from the dinner table with the feeling that you ate more than you really wanted — perhaps just a *little* too much — but just enough to make you feel uncomfortably full?

If that feeling of being stuffed to the gills is a familiar one, you need to restructure your mealtime eating habits.

If you usually feel satisfied, but not stuffed — except after a holiday feast — mealtime probably isn't your problem.

On the other hand, if you seldom feel really satisfied after eating a meal, you probably *do* have a major mealtime problem — one which might be worse than feeling stuffed, because it's encouraging the likelihood of late-night binges.

You might think that the purely subjective feeling you have upon getting up from the table is a poor way to judge whether or not you have eaten too much, but in truth it's probably the best way. The idea that someone on a reducing diet ought to eat a dinner consisting of precisely 500 or 700 calories is simply ridiculous. Why should a 220-pound man be satisfied or nourished by the same meal prescribed for a 165-pound man? Yet, that is the approach traditionally taken in diet plans, and is another reason why they almost always fail.

Eating a meal, particularly dinner, is a very special kind of behavior. If you've been reading diet plans, I want you to forget all about them right now, because they are going to hinder you, not help you. The concept underlying nearly all these plans is that meal-eating is simply the episodic ingestion of nutrients — something like a layman's version of intravenous feeding. Just pour less food down the tubes, this approach recommends, and you will lose weight. Some dieticians who share this belief don't tell you exactly how many calories you ought to eat at a meal, but simply recommend that you "cut down the portions." Well, that's a perfectly logical statement, but it's about as helpful as telling a businessman that the path to success lies in boosting his profit margins. He already knows that. And you know you ought to be cutting down your portions. The trick is *how.*

The most important thing to understand about dinner time, I think, is that eating a meal is a *ritual,* perhaps the most basic ritual of human life. It's something you have done tens of thousands of times. Each of us brings to the occasion all sorts of deeply ingrained habits and expectations. For many of us, dinner time is also an important social occasion. It may be the only time that the family gets together as a unit to share an activity. If that's the case, anger or frustration that may have been building all day may suddenly erupt at the table. Likewise, feelings of friendship and love that may be bottled up during the rest of the day may suddenly find expression over meat and potatoes.

The moral is that if we pretend dinner time is nothing but shoveling food into our mouths in a kind of social vacuum, all that energy endemic to the mealtime ritual is going to rapidly overwhelm our best intentions and drown them in a bowl of gravy. But if we understand something about that ritualistic energy, and plan our changes accordingly, we may discover that it really isn't that difficult to achieve success — right from the very first day.

Mealtime actually begins long before somebody says "Dinner is ready!" Let's consider the following true example:

Julia summons her husband and children to the table. The main course is scallops, which both Julia and her husband enjoy greatly. But trouble starts fast. Because scallops were so expensive, Julia was only able to buy a small amount. As soon as her husband sees the skimpy portion on his plate, he gets a frustrated feeling, and lets Julia know about it. That makes Julia feel very distressed, so she immediately goes into the refrigerator and comes out with all sorts of leftovers which she piles in front of her husband as a kind of testimony to the fact that she still loves him. She also gives her husband several of her scallops, which gives *her* a ticket to dive into the leftovers, too. Twenty minutes later, both of their stomachs are bursting with scallops, vegetables, potato salad, and cold beef sandwiches. Still trying to make up for a botched meal, Julia gives her husband an especially large helping of dessert. And to make herself feel better, has some extra pie, too. . . . Only instead of feeling better, she feels worse.

There are innumerable variations on that theme. But what they all boil down to is that the unstructured meal easily becomes an occasion to plunder the refrigerator and pillage the pantry in a desperate attempt to put something on the table that is going to feel like dinner. Almost invariably, it's a case of overkill. And "kill" is probably the right word. Because what we're doing amounts to killing the appetite by brute force, rather than satisfying it with the kind of careful, loving attention our bodies deserve.

A disorganized meal is bad not only because it can lead to too much food being put on the table. When there is no structure or "theme" to a meal, it actually *takes* more food, more calories, to give us that sense of satisfaction we desire. Recall how much you had to eat to feel satisfied the last time you had a really fine and attractively served meal. Compare that to the amount you had to eat to reach satisfaction the last time you sat down (or stood up) to a chaotic kind of potluck meal. Somehow, if it doesn't seem like a "real dinner," you may find yourself eating excessive amounts of food simply to convince yourself that you really *had* dinner.

Learn to structure your meal. Our first principle, then, is: *Always know what you're going to have for dinner well before you begin preparing a meal.* If you get into the habit of doing that, there will be no pressing need to measure portions, count calories, or forego your favorite foods. When you plan your meals, eating appropriate portions will follow naturally.

Planning a meal begins at the kitchen table — not with knife and fork but with pencil and paper. For most people, planning meals about a week in advance works best. Whether you're going to be trying some new recipes, relying on family favorites, or both, it's extremely helpful to have the actual list of ingredients right in front of you. It's worth double-checking to make sure that you have all the appropriate condiments for each recipe or meal; Parmesan cheese for the pasta, lemon for the fish, yogurt for the baked potato, and so forth. Herbs, spices, and condiments help give food the quality of being a "meal," which is exactly the quality that we're striving for.

Principle Number Two: *Try to buy only as much food as will fit into your planned menus.* There are two ways to do this: one is to make every effort not to buy excessive amounts of food in the first place, and the other is to learn how to use leftovers in a creative but planned manner. If you're the kind of person who knows how to turn leftovers into a good lunch or dinner, you have a definite advantage here. If not, you can either ask friends for tips, buy some recipe books, or be especially diligent when making your purchases. That may mean, for instance, going a little out of your way to buy meat from a butcher instead of the supermarket, in order to get the portions you really want. Instead of buying a whole chicken, you may want to buy a couple of split breasts or some legs. A butcher will usually give you exactly the amount of ground beef you want and it's easy to store leftovers, raw or cooked, for future use. You may also want to emphasize nonmeat items in your diet because many are easily stored and conveniently portionable: rice, bulgur, noodles, beans, and potatoes.

It's interesting that just as the easily stored and portioned foods mentioned above are high in nutrition and low in fat, foods which can create real leftover problems tend to be high in fat or calories: pork roasts, spareribs, and all sorts of cakes, pies, and special desserts. The biggest trouble with a chocolate cake, for instance, is not so much the calories in one piece, but the difficulty so many of us have keeping the leftover portion for later use. That "later use" too often turns out to be three hours after you've had your first serving.

Principle Number Three: *Don't put more on the table than you want to eat at that meal.* In the case of the chocolate cake mentioned before, the sensible thing to do is to cut out one large piece that can be divided into a reasonable portion for everyone at the table and then wrap and store the remainder. Putting the rest of that cake in the freezer may also be a good idea, so you won't have to "worry" that it will go bad unless you polish it off. Some cooks enjoy bringing a large roast or casserole to the table because it looks very impressive. But if experience tells you that all that food sitting on the table is going to create a desire to eat more than you really want, do the carving or serving on the kitchen counter top and then store the rest before eating. An alternative would be to put the whole dish on the table, serve the food, then immediately remove what's left and store it. If you're really hungry, you can always get more, and there's nothing at all wrong with doing that. *All you're trying to do is structure your dinner in such a way as to encourage a pattern of eating based on real hunger, instead of habit, impulse, and the plate-cleaning syndrome.* Remember: food sitting on the table during a meal is more likely to be consumed "unconsciously" than in any other situation.

Principle Number Four: *Take away leftovers and unfinished*

dinners as soon as possible, for storage or disposal. This principle is simply the follow-through to the previous one. If there's anything more apt to be eaten unconsciously than extra food sitting on the table at dinner time, it's extra food sitting on your *plate* after you've finished your main bout of eating. Somehow, there's always that extra potato, a few extra tablespoons of gravy, that piece of bread, or half of Jimmy's dinner that mysteriously winds up on your own plate. The place for that extra food is the refrigerator, the bread box — or the garbage can if need be. If it feels like it's a shame not to "do something" with that good food, just stop for a moment and picture what that "good food" is going to look like on your neck and thighs. Do you really want to use your body as a kind of warehouse or silo? If not, get busy and clean off that table!

Sidetrack your eating momentum. The fifth and last principle is really a comprehensive set of skills that I call: *Learn to sidetrack your eating momentum.*

Through observation of my own eating habits and questioning workshop participants, it became clear to me that a considerable amount of overeating that takes place at dinner time is the result of a kind of almost mindless momentum that builds up rapidly and doesn't grind to a halt until you've eaten *much* more than you need, *considerably* more than you really wanted, and just enough to make you feel like every cell in your body has been stuffed full of food. Many of us, I'm sure, astonish ourselves with our ability to eat large bowls of soup, buttered rolls, heaping plates of salad, and big chunks of meat without putting the brakes on that momentum. Often, that eating drive doesn't sputter to a halt until we sneak pieces of food from serving dishes even as we carry them to the refrigerator to be stored.

Yet, 15 minutes later, we feel so overfed that we realize it wasn't true hunger that made us eat all that extra food. It was nothing but sheer *eating momentum.*

The most dangerous — and ineffective — way to stop something with a lot of momentum behind it, whether it's a locomotive or your appetite, is to stand in front of it and let it plow into you. When we do that with a locomotive, it's called suicide; when we do it with eating momentum, it's called willpower.

The right way, the effective way, of extracting the dangerous momentum from an onrushing object is to sidetrack it: divert its energy off on a tangent, a safe tangent, where it can either run out of steam naturally or be braked in a variety of ways until it reaches a manageable energy level.

What that means at the dinner table is that rather than merely giving ourselves small portions of food and then jumping up from the table in a spasm of willpower, we're going to reengineer our dinner ritual, lay down some new tracks as it were, so that we can control the momentum that keeps us eating past the point where we've had enough.

The single, most important cause of uncontrollable eating momentum is the failure of our nervous systems to throw our appetites into neutral when our stomachs have received an appropriate amount of food. How often have you finished eating, not feeling particularly stuffed, only to feel positively sluggish and bloated 20 or 30 minutes later? That's the failure I'm referring to, although "failure" might not be the right word.

It would be nice, wouldn't it, if our stomachs and the nerve centers with which they communicate could give us what computer people call "real-time feedback" a few seconds after we swallowed every morsel of food. That way, we would know — *and feel* — exactly how far along we were in the process of meeting our metabolic needs, and when they were satisfied, our appetites would instantly and automatically be thrown into neutral.

But as we all know, that doesn't happen. And for good reason. Our eating control system, by which I refer to the whole complex of organs, nerves, and chemical substances which regulate appetite, is too smart to be caught playing that instant feedback game. Were it to do that, we would probably all be stumbling around in a state of severe malnutrition, because every time we ate a few pieces of fruit or some bulky, low-calorie vegetables, or drank two glasses of water, we'd feel as though we'd just eaten a complete meal.

What our appetite control system wants to do before signaling us that it's time to quit is *analyze* what we've eaten. Find out if it contains enough real nourishment. And that takes some time, because food first has to be processed by stomach acids, moved through the pyloric valve into the small intestine, and then absorbed — at least partially — into the system. At that point, the control system knows what we've eaten and is prepared to begin downshifting our jaw muscles. Scientists who have studied this process say that it takes about 20 to 25 minutes for this process to occur — and those 20 minutes become a critical factor in learning to sidetrack your eating momentum.

Actually, some people, particularly children and very slender adults, seem to respond to food more quickly than that, and experience the sensation of fullness within five or ten minutes after they begin eating. My belief is that that greater sensitivity is a natural gift many of us lose — along with other natural sensitivities — as we grow older and become accustomed to responding more to external cues than to our own bodies and spirits. In fact, it's my experience that as you begin to control your eating, and begin slowly to lose weight, some of that sensitivity returns. If after dieting for a while, you've said that "my stomach seems to have shrunk," what you're experiencing, I believe, is the return of that sensitivity.

But until such time as your appetite control system may learn to respond more quickly, you have to live with the reality of that 20-minute delay.

The first thing to do is to make the first item on the dinner menu a dish which contains both protein and fat. Those two substances are exactly what thc appetite control system wants to find before braking our appetites. Apparently, it realizes that if protein and fat are being absorbed, almost inevitably there will be a sufficiency of calories, vitamins, and minerals coming in along with them. That is not always the case, but that's the way the system seems to work, according to current knowledge. By eating protein and fat at the beginning of the meal, then, what you're doing is immediately sending those two substances on their way to the appetite control system, so that your eating momentum doesn't continue for any longer than it has to.

Consider, for a moment, the alternative. You sit down to dinner, telling yourself that you don't want second helpings of meat and potatoes and that you're going to achieve that goal by stuffing yourself with sheer bulk. So first, you drink a glass of water, then a big bowl of bouillon, and then plow through an enormous bowl of salad. But the minute you've finished the salad, your appetite for some inexplicable reason seems to be greater than ever, and you go tearing into your steak and potatoes with a vengeance. At least, that's what's happened to me many times, and diet workshop participants report similar experiences. What apparently is happening is that all that soup and salad isn't doing much other than signaling to your digestive system that a big meal is on its way. There is so little protein and fat in traditional early-meal items such as water, clear broth, wine, and salad that the appetite continues raging, demanding some "real food."

One simple way to hasten the onset of a feeling of fullness is to eat the main course of your dinner as soon as you sit down. No matter what it is, it's likely to have more protein and fat than appetizers, vegetables, or even desserts. An alternative is to have a bowl of soup that has some solid protein in it, like clam chowder or a chunky chicken soup. Interestingly, beginning the meal with just such a hearty soup is a common practice in many cultures. Another traditional ethnic dish is chopped liver, also high in both protein and fat. Antipasto, with its meats and cheeses and oil, also fills the bill — although it may *over*-fill the bill.

As for your large salad and your cantaloupe wedges, save them for later, something like a kind of dessert. As you are eating your main course, you can keep in mind that you still have the salad or maybe even some soup coming, so if it feels as though you aren't quite filled when you're done eating that main dish, have no fear, because there is still plenty of munching ahead of you. Then, by the time you finish your soup and salad, the protein and fat from your main course should begin to be absorbed and bring down the curtain on the show. And while you're waiting for that to happen, if you have extra helpings of salad, there's no harm done.

More ways to sidetrack your eating momentum. Many if not most people who eat too much at a meal also eat too rapidly. Naturally, the faster you eat, the more you can put away before your appetite control system has a chance to swing into action. There is also a psychological component here, because many people who eat too rapidly are barely conscious that they're eating. Their attention is focused on a newspaper or a heavy conversation. Many people eat while they're watching TV. Since your brain is an integral part of your appetite control system, why not let it in on the fact that you're eating dinner?

Just *how* slowly you ought to eat is difficult to say. Probably the best thing to do is experiment with various speeds. You can begin by trying to eat approximately 50 percent slower than you do now — assuming that you're a fast eater. First, tell yourself, "I'm going to eat dinner now." Then look at the food on your plate very carefully. Describe it to yourself. When you take your first bite of something, put down your silverware and chew your food slowly and thoroughly, so that you experience its flavor, texture, and aroma. Take another forkful of food only after you have thoroughly savored and swallowed your first. Put down your silverware again, lean back in your chair, and enjoy yourself. *Be aware that eating is one of the most important things you do, and that it's perfectly reasonable to eat in a slow and thoughtful manner.* Most people also find eating quite enjoyable, so why eat as fast as you can? Your new way of eating will not only make the experience last longer, but will make it more enjoyable because you'll be much more in touch with the experience of eating — as opposed to unconsciously shoveling food into your mouth.

If you want to, you can experiment with techniques which *really* slow down eating. If you're right-handed, hold your fork in your left hand. Chew each mouthful of food 50 times. Wait 15 seconds between mouthfuls. Try chewing your food in slow motion, as if it were the last morsel of food you were ever going to have in your life. If dinner comes in different courses, try waiting five minutes between each course. Or plan your meal so that it's served that way. In between courses, get up from the table and prepare the next course, or do something else. Don't keep sitting at the table or you'll become terribly impatient.

Some of these techniques may sound a little unnatural, but I'm not so sure they are. I vividly remember watching a big Siberian tiger at the Philadelphia Zoo just before feeding time. When the feeding man came in with a can of raw meat, all the big cats began to growl and leap around their cages. Finally it was the tiger's turn to be thrown a big chunk of horse meat. I expected him to swallow the thing practically whole. But just the opposite happened. He picked up his dinner in his jaws, walked over to the middle of his cage, eased himself down into a comfortable position, and proceeded to make love to that hunk of horse meat. He licked it, nibbled it, sniffed it, and finally began chewing it, very slowly, in the corner of his mouth. Now there's somebody who *enjoys* his dinner!

I confess that I don't lick my meat, but if eating like that is good enough for a Siberian tiger, it can't be all that unnatural.

Robert Rodale, the editor of *Prevention* magazine, believes that people can help themselves to lose weight by eating foods that require more jaw movements to chew. "Meals of soft food are swallowed too quickly," he explains. "You take in too many calories too quickly, without realizing how much you have eaten."

His favorite food — and possibly a useful tool for dieters — is a hard, homemade corn cracker* (also called a corn pone) that is cheap, tastes good, and must be chewed thoroughly before being swallowed.

"One time I counted the number of times I chewed each bite of corn cracker," he said. "I was surprised to find that 40 chews were necessary to get the corn in a smooth enough consistency to be swallowed. Then I gave some of the corn meal crackers to other people and watched how many times they chewed before swallowing each bite. Nobody could get a bite down with fewer than 40 chews."

Possibly the vigorous exercising of jaw muscles signals the appetite control system that a person has had enough to eat. At least, that's the theory behind the hard-food dieting idea.

Another technique that can help slow down your eating momentum is to change the *time* that you eat dinner. Many of our workshop participants said that if they ate immediately upon coming home from work, their appetites seemed to be particularly ravenous. Ironically, several said that if they waited an hour or two to have dinner, they felt much less hungry. That may not seem to make much sense, but if you think about it, you may find that when you return from a day's work, your "appetite" at that moment is being fueled by tension built up during the day, and probably the tension involved in driving home. What seems to be happening is that as soon as you leave work, you know that the next thing on the agenda is to eat, and the expectation of that meal keeps building up until you get to the kitchen. Often, the eagerness to eat is so great that you begin eating within seconds of entering your house. But what's driving you at that moment is not true hunger, but a pattern of habit, expectation, and tension.

One of our workshop participants had the same experience I did: when she delayed dinner for about two hours — filling that time with carefully planned activities such as a walk and household chores — she found that her hunger had greatly abated. Although you may never have tried that technique, you may have experienced the results just the same. Did you ever "lose your appetite" because a meal habitually eaten at a certain time was delayed for half an hour or more?

---

* Robert Rodale's recipe for corn crackers: Preheat oven to 350°. Combine 3 cups of cornmeal and ¼ cup of sesame seeds in a large bowl. Stir in ½ cup of corn oil and 1½ cups of boiling water, adding just enough additional water to form a stiff batter. Allow batter to cool. With your hands oiled, form flat cakes, and place on an oiled cookie sheet. Bake for about 40 minutes.

If your motive was purely hunger, that wouldn't happen. The edge was taken off your appetite simply because a long-standing habit pattern had suddenly been broken.

A variation of that approach is to try making lunch your main meal instead of dinner. For the last few months, that's what I've been doing, and it seems to be working well. Because I eat lunch out, there is no opportunity to raid the pantry. Then, at dinner time, I have something light, like melon and cottage cheese. (On this regimen, I discovered that my energy level for evening work kept to a much more even keel.)

No matter how large your dinner, many people still have a desire for something sweet before leaving the table. That is nothing more than sheer habit, like wanting a cigarette after a meal, and with a little effort, the desire will abate. By eating a large salad at the end of your meal, most of the battle will be won, because habitually you don't eat sweets right after a salad. There may also be something to the theory that strongly flavored foods like meats and rich sauces encourage the desire for something sweet immediately afterward, to balance the taste buds, perhaps. Finishing the meal with something relatively bland, like salad, or even some bread, will help. Robert Rodale says his corn crackers not only satisfy his jaw muscles, but have a nut-like flavor that cleanses the palate after a meal, and wipes away stronger flavor sensations that sometimes cause people to want to keep eating. Eating a few nuts — or corn pones — at the end of a meal is a low-calorie way to signal a stop to the eating process. Perhaps that's the origin of the phrase "from soup to nuts."

What works for me is a cup of unsweetened peppermint tea which also leaves the mouth feeling clean and satisfied. If you like an occasional cup of tea or coffee, it's a good idea to have one already brewed and waiting so that you can immediately enjoy it when you're done eating. You will find that in a short time, you will lay down a new habit pattern, so that the drinking of your herb tea or munching of your corn pone becomes a powerful signaling device to your system that the meal has come to a conclusion.

However you conclude your meal, you should tell yourself: "This is the way I'm *supposed* to feel. Not stuffed, but satisfied. This feeling is really much better than being stuffed and sluggish. Fifteen minutes from now I'll feel even more satisfied than I am now. So why should I clog up my body's machinery with too much food?"

At that point, leave the table and immediately begin some purposeful activity. Whether it's washing the dishes or reading a book, taking your dog for a walk or sewing, the idea is that you should *know* what you're going to do, so that you don't simply sit at the table for lack of anything better to do.

If others are still at the table and you want to enjoy their company, take away your own plate, wash your hands, and then return to the table. Or carry on a conversation while you do the dishes at the sink. One of the best techniques for women is to return to the table with some knitting, because no one is going to eat unconsciously while they're knitting. If you enjoy playing a musical instrument, right after dinner is a fine time to practice. An evening chess game immediately after dinner, right at the cleaned-off table, is another good idea.

The dangerous art of skipping meals. Several people in our workshop asked if it is a good idea to skip meals to save calories. My answer was that skipping meals is probably the worst thing you can do on your new eating program. But does that mean, they asked, that you should eat dinner even when you aren't hungry, or only feel like a light bite? Hmmm . . . a good question!

First, let's see what typically happens when you try to skip a meal. I say "typically" because I used to try it often myself, and so did some of our workshop participants.

Dinner time rolls around — let's say half-past six — and for some reason you aren't quite as hungry as you usually are. Suddenly you get the idea that maybe you'll just skip dinner. Tomorrow it will be time to weigh yourself, so why not take one last good whack at your flab? By seven you've forgotten all about dinner and at eight you're still feeling no pain. However, at about half-past eight, you begin to feel an ominous rumbling down below. Slowly, over the next hour, a yawning chasm seems to be opening in your belly. Desperately, you throw yourself into different activities to try to forget your hunger. But at ten o'clock you can't stand it anymore, so you figure you'll just give that chasm some first aid by stuffing it with a peanut butter sandwich. One minute later, the peanut butter sandwich is gone but not the chasm. Amazing how stomach chasms just love to swallow peanut butter sandwiches! Should you eat another one? Well, what the heck, you didn't have dinner, anyway, so. . . . Just a few minutes later, you're still standing in front of the refrigerator, your appetite greater than ever. Then your spouse comes along and asks if you would like your dinner heated up. Well, just a little, you answer. Naturally, just about everything that's left gets heated up, and five minutes later you sit down and eat a dinner as large as you would have eaten at half-past six. In fact, all you leave is the vegetables.

Sound familiar? It used to happen to me all the time. Finally, after maybe the tenth repeat, it dawned on me that these futile attempts to skip dinner were resulting only in my eating several hundred calories *more* than I would have if I hadn't tried to skip a meal. Without fail, I would become ravenously hungry at about ten or eleven o'clock at night, and begin eating little bits of almost anything, downing the food so fast I hardly tasted it or knew what it was. And if something inside me would say "I can't believe you're doing this!" something else would say "But I didn't eat dinner! I *need* something to eat!"

Although there are legitimate reasons for skipping meals, doing so as a technique to lose weight is not one of them. The combination of a drastic departure from routine plus almost inevitable feelings of deprivation constitute a catastrophic combination. The feeling that your appetite is not quite all that it could be is no better as a reason to try skipping a meal. If it's convenient, you can *delay* your meal, but if you try to skip it, your appetite will almost surely return in a few hours and if you don't have a planned meal ready, you might find yourself going on an eating rampage.

But perhaps you ate a very large lunch. Or perhaps you're too tired to eat. To evaluate the condition of your hunger, try to vividly imagine yourself eating dinner and see what it feels like. If it turns you off completely, maybe you really don't have an appetite. Still, plan what you *are* going to eat should your appetite suddenly return. "Lost" appetites have been known to be found at one o'clock in the morning!

Having said all that, there are still a few — *very* few — occasions when not eating a planned meal is reasonable. When I know that I'm going out to a good restaurant for dinner, I almost never eat lunch. That permits me to indulge in the occasional luxury of wine and a sumptuous dessert without exceeding my caloric needs for that day. But I don't necessarily recommend that for everyone. Some people simply cannot handle the results of a skipped meal, which may include severe hunger pangs, irritability, plummeting blood sugar levels, even a headache. Other people should avoid skipping meals because they practically go berserk when they finally do decide to eat. For those of you who *are* able to skip a meal in anticipation of an unusually large one later, I would urge that the meal skipped be the one *before* the large one. I'd also urge that, as a rule, dinner should not be skipped under any circumstances. Hunger pangs that attack late at night are the most difficult to deal with.

Aside from the anticipation of a feast, or a trip to an amusement park where there's a lot of snacks that you want to indulge in, there are remarkably few legitimate reasons for skipping meals. I sometimes skip meals when I'm traveling because airplane and airport food is not much to my liking. If I'm going to skip dinner, though, I always try to make sure that I go to bed early, because I know that if I'm awake past eleven, I'm going to become ravenous.

To conclude this chapter, I'd like to make two points. First, while it may sound a little unnatural to pay so much attention to something as mundane as a meal, remember that eating is one of the most basic and important rituals of life. Therefore, it's both logical and perfectly natural to give it a great amount of thought.

Second, modifications in mealtime behavior are a process of trial and error, of experimentation, of self-discovery and ongoing health improvement. Expect many of the things you try not to work out exactly right. But learn from them. It may take weeks, or even months until you feel comfortable with a new set of mealtime eating habits. But keep trying — not with your willpower, but with your thinking, planning, and experimenting. Those are the tools that are going to work for you. Don't expect or even try for radical changes. When all's said and done, I would consider your new eating pattern to be highly successful if it results in the daily saving of 100 calories, which is no more than a single piece of bread dipped in a little gravy. Combine that saving with just 100 calories less from snacking, and another 150 calories expended on a half-hour of walking, and you will lose 25 pounds. I'll explain that arithmetic in the next chapter; right now, just be assured that small, thoughtful changes in your routine can add up to big changes. And a smaller you.

9

The New Math of Realistic Weight Loss

We haven't said much so far about calories per se. That's because I wanted to emphasize the fact that the path to success is not so much a way of dieting as a way of eating. A new, more natural and healthful way of eating that will let you lose weight, yes, but much more important, maintain your ideal weight once you have reached it.

Having made this point, it's now time to talk about calories and what they mean. Doing so will enable you to visualize the effect that changes in eating habits are going to have on your waistline. We will also take advantage of this discussion of calories to review some of the eating techniques we've already learned, and to introduce some new ones.

I suppose the most basic fact is that when you eat 3,000 calories which are not burned up by your metabolic needs or exercise, you will gain one pound of fat. Perhaps you have read that the consumption of 3,500 calories is required to create one pound of fat. That's the figure that is generally used. But like so much else that's published about weight control, even that simple statement is wrong. It's true that 3,500 calories can lead to the formation of one pound of fat, but only *theoretically*. Because as soon as you begin depositing fat in your body, you begin to retain water. Even the cells in which the fat is enveloped have to gain weight to take care of the extra burden. The result is that — largely because of water retention — you only have to consume about 2,950 calories to add one pound of excess weight to your body. For the sake of convenience, let's say 3,000 calories.

If you overeat by 100 calories a day, then, you will gain 1 pound in about 30 days.

If you eat 100 calories *less* than you require to meet your needs, you will *lose* 1 pound in one month.

But suppose you go on eating those 100 extra calories a day not for one month, but for a year. Will you gain 12 pounds? Would you gain 240 pounds in 20 years? Gratefully, no; weight gain doesn't work that way.

When you have gained 1 extra pound of fat, you have at that point increased the number of calories you are automatically burning up each day by 14. That's the approximate number of calories that are required to keep that pound of fat at body temperature, care for its metabolic needs, and carry it around all day long. When you have gained 10 pounds, you will be burning up an additional 140 calories. If you are 50 pounds overweight, you will be burning up some 700 calories a day more than if you were at your ideal weight. Obviously, then, if you are eating 100 calories a day more than you required at the beginning, and your exercise output remains the same, you will not gain 12 pounds in one year. By the time you add 7 pounds, your daily fuel requirement will have been upped by 98 calories — just about enough to offset those extra 100 calories perfectly. Assuming that you go on doing everything just the way you have been, your weight will stay at that point — 7 pounds heavier.

That gives us a formula by which we can predict the weight gain that will be produced by a given number of extra calories. Simply divide the number of additional calories by 14, and you have the number of pounds at which your weight will stabilize after a period of gain. Eat 140 calories a day too much, and you will gain ten pounds — and keep it.

That also explains why the pattern of weight gain is usually to put on quite a few pounds at the beginning of the gaining cycle, and then progressively fewer. As the pounds add up, they burn calories, and the fattening effect of the caloric overshoot slows down.

It's important to realize that this cycle of weight gain can be initiated by a decrease in exercise as well as an increase in food. If you decrease the number of calories you are putting out in exercise each day by 100 — something which happens to many of us at some point in our 20s — your requirement for calories to maintain your weight at an even level is reduced by 100. If you go on eating just as you were before, you will be consuming 100 calories too many. Some people would say that the real trouble is not that you are eating too much, but that you are exercising too little. But the net effect is exactly the same. When you cut back in your energy output by 100 calories a day, you will — eating the same food you were before — gain 7 pounds. Ordinarily, most of us begin to slow down at about the time we get married, but slow down even more as we grow older. That explains why our weight gain doesn't stop at 5 or 10 pounds, but keeps on increasing. If, by the time we reach 45, for example, we have cut back our energy output by an average of 300 calories a day, we'll be carrying around an additional 21 pounds of fat. Sometimes, as we grow older, we reduce the number of calories we eat. In that case, if the same 45-year-old person were eating 100 calories a day less than he or she was before the period of weight gain, he would be carrying around only 14 extra pounds of fat.

It's easy to turn this formula around and discover what effect *losing* weight has on calorie consumption. For each pound of fat you lose, you reduce the number of calories you are automatically burning by 14. After you have lost 10 pounds, your daily "burn rate" will have been reduced by 140 calories.

Therefore, if you cut back your eating by 100 calories a day (or increase your exercise by 100 calories a day) you will, over a period of months, lose 7 pounds. Weight loss will be greatest during the first month, and progressively slower as you lose weight. After having lost 7 pounds, your actual requirement for food will be 100 calories less, so your input will exactly balance your output. If you want to know what the ultimate effect will be of eating 150 fewer calories a day, and getting 150 calories worth of additional exercise each day, add them together and divide the total by 14. The answer is about 21 pounds. It would be exactly the same if, instead of reducing your food intake and exercising as well, you simply reduced your food intake by 300 calories a day.

The 300 Plan. Which brings us to a question that eventually comes up for some readers. Namely, just *how many* calories is it reasonable to remove from your diet?

"I've been following your approach, and becoming more conscious of how and why I'm eating," Warren said. "But I feel a little uneasy about it because I'm not really sure if what I'm cutting out of my diet is a reasonable amount. Maybe it's even too much."

For people like Warren, who feel more comfortable with some additional guidance, I have come up with what I call the 300 Plan. This plan suggests that 300 calories a day is a good average figure of calorie reduction to aim for, at least during the first few months of reducing. It also helps locate the most "vulnerable" 300 calories in a diet, and then suggests ways by which they can be done away with in a relatively harmless fashion.

Some people do not need this guidance, and there is nothing terribly special about the figure of 300 calories. I have chosen that as an average figure to aim for because experience shows that most people can cut that much out of their daily food intake without feeling hungry, deprived, or weak. It's also enough of a reduction to produce a loss of 21 pounds. However, my advice is to *combine* this cutback of 300 calories of food with an *increase* of about 200 calories worth of exercise — equivalent to about 45 minutes of walking. That combined approach will produce a deficit of some 500 calories a day, producing a weight loss of about 5 pounds the first month, and slightly but progressively less each succeeding month, with the net effect being a loss of 35 pounds.

What if you want to lose *more* than 35 pounds? What then? That's a good question, and as a matter of fact it came up just yesterday, when I contacted a young woman who was one of the more diligent members of a workshop which concluded about six months ago. By the end of the workshop, she said, she had in fact lost exactly 35 pounds (sounds like I made it up, but it's true!). She also said she has had "no trouble" keeping that weight off. However, she hasn't been able to lose any more weight, and she still wants to lose about another 20 pounds. She was puzzled, too, because she didn't understand why her weight loss didn't continue.

I explained to her that having lost 35 pounds, she was now burning some 490 calories a day less than she was when she began the program. In other words, she had reached the point at which less food and more exercise (amounting to 500 calories a day) were exactly balancing the caloric needs of her new, lower weight.

I went on to advise her that she should be very aware of the fact that she is now, very literally, *a new person.* That while a reduction of 300 calories a day was appropriate for her a year ago, her needs are so much smaller now, and her true hunger so much less, that it would be not only appropriate, but relatively easy, to decrease her caloric input still more. I suggested that she reduce her daily calorie total by about 100 a day to start with, and when she felt quite comfortable with that, to cut out 100 more. At the same time, I suggested she try for more exercise, which would burn up about another 100 calories a day. (In fact, she'd just joined a health spa.) Following that plan, the last 20 pounds of her unwanted fat would inevitably fall away.

It's easy to modify the principles of the 300 Plan so that it *eventually* becomes a 400 Plan or a 500 Plan. Remember, after losing 21 pounds on the 300 Plan (or more if you're exercising), you have become a new person. It is perfectly reasonable and logical for you to cut back your food intake at that point. And to keep reducing it, *gradually,* until you reach the point where you are at your ideal weight, and your losing has come to a natural end.

And what happens at that point? Nothing! You just keep on doing exactly as you have been, following your new habits. There is no "diet" to go off. You completely avoid the trap that destroys people who lose a lot of weight following a 1,200-calorie diet, and then, when they reach their target weight, simply revert to eating the way they were before. Instead, you change nothing, realizing that you have engineered for yourself a new way of eating and living that is perfectly designed to maintain your ideal weight.

It may have struck you that weight loss in this approach is not produced at blinding speed. But that's a plus, not a minus. Any expert in weight reduction will tell you that the faster weight comes off, the faster it comes back. Both your body and your behavior *need* that time in order to become totally accustomed to new eating patterns. So, although it may sound a little strange, it's important to realize that *it is better to lose weight slowly than rapidly.* We already know that our problem is not losing weight, anyway, but keeping it off, and your chances of maintaining your new weight will be enormously greater if you lose your weight over a period of, say, one year, rather than three months.

You will be much better off aiming for a very modest reduction of calories at first, and then gradually increasing it, rather than aiming for too great an initial decrease. If there is any optimal rate of weight loss, my estimate is that it would be in the vicinity of 3 pounds a month if you're doing it by reduced food intake alone, and about 5 pounds a month if you're combining the dietary approach with exercise. *That means a weight reduction of anywhere between 36 and 60 pounds in a year's time.* More important, it means weight reduction that's much more likely to be *permanent.*

The 300 Plan in action. Now let's see what removing 300 calories a day actually looks like, and feels like.

Keep in mind that the food we are listing here is that which is habitually or typically part of your daily diet, and that you are *not* going to eat.

The second important point is that the foods selected for these daily deductions are chosen not simply because they happen to add up to 300 calories, but because they fall into one or more of the following categories:

- Junk foods which contribute nothing to your well-being.
- Foods which are typically consumed as snacks (recreational eating).
- Foods which can be divided in such a way that you can eat less of them without feeling deprived.
- Foods which are consumed as second helpings (often because of the sheer momentum of rapid eating or permitting them to sit on the table after the meal has been completed).
- Foods that don't give you a great sense of satisfaction.

	Calories
One-half cup beef hash	200
One can ginger ale	113
Total	313

In the first example, the half-cup of beef hash represents a second helping which is habitually eaten but is now not even put on the table. The can of ginger ale, consumed largely for its amusement value, has been pushed out of the picture by good spring water, club soda, or coffee. Even if a teaspoon of sugar were added to the coffee, the total saving for the day would still be 300 calories.

	Calories
One-half piece buttered toast w/jelly	70
One tablespoon Russian dressing	75
One Coke	144
One very small cheese cracker (145 per pound)	15
Total	304

This example, like most of the others we'll be giving, is arranged in the approximate order that these food items typically appear in the daily diet. Let's say that this individual typically breakfasts on a glass of orange juice, one scrambled egg, one piece of buttered toast with jelly, and a cup of coffee. He decides to try eating half that piece of toast and discovers that he can do it without feeling hungry or deprived. He might have left off the jelly and eaten the entire piece of buttered toast and saved almost as many calories, but when he tried that, he found that without the jelly, he *did* feel unsatisfied.

He then went on to eat his usual lunch, but at dinner, when he typically used two tablespoons of Russian dressing on his salad, he cut out one of those tablespoons by the simple expedient of tossing the salad with the dressing in a big bowl. After dinner, he typically would have a bottle of Coke and a handful of cheese crackers; now he has half a cup of coffee and one or two fewer cheese crackers. And he's very careful about not eating those crackers from the box, but rather removing the exact number that he wants to eat and then putting the box in the back of the pantry.

	Calories
One pat of butter	36
One-half tablespoon mayonnaise	50
Five potato chips	55
One-third cup pork and beans	104
One dozen shelled, roasted peanuts	60
Total	305

This man hasn't changed his breakfast. His first deduction comes at lunch, when he tells the waiter at his favorite restaurant that he'd like the cook to go easy on the mayonnaise on his turkey sandwich, and to hold the potato chips. At dinner, he spreads only a little butter on his bread and his vegetables (using prewarmed butter that will spread thinly) and forgoes the second helping of pork and beans. Later, at nine o'clock, he skips his usual handful of salted nuts.

		Calories
One-half piece buttered toast		55
One large forkful of apple pie		50
Two thin pretzels		70
One slice pizza		153
	Total	328

Sally lives with family members who typically have pie after almost every meal. Although she "doesn't eat any herself," she does take one forkful which "can't hurt." When she finds out that it *does* hurt when she does it three times a week, she gives up this habit. It so happens that this is a Friday night, when she and her husband typically go out and split a pizza. Usually, her husband will have five pieces, while she has three. After thinking about it, she realizes that after eating two, she's perfectly satisfied and that in fact, that third piece makes her feel uncomfortable. So she decides to "trash her fat" and leave the piece on the pizza pan whether her husband eats it or not.

		Calories
One slice bacon		43
Two cheese-peanut butter cracker "sandwiches"		70
Three large prunes		60
One-half cup Jell-o		71
Six cashews		68
	Total	312

This woman eats a fairly substantial breakfast, so one less slice of bacon isn't going to interfere seriously with her normal eating pattern. After that, she accomplishes everything she needs to in the way of calorie reduction simply by removing a few snacks. Notice, incidentally, how many calories there are in a couple of peanut butter and cheese crackers!

	Calories
One-half cup coleslaw (made with mayonnaise)	85
One slice American cheese	105
One piece bologna	57
One-quarter cup ice cream	64
One rye wafer	20
Total	331

Here's a person who does not eat a great deal of junk food or even many desserts, except for a half-cup of ice cream every night at about eleven o'clock. Most of the overeating seems to be in the afternoon. The deductions came with the simple expedients of a serving of coleslaw only half as large as usual, and eating a sandwich made with only one piece of cheese and two pieces of bologna, rather than two pieces of cheese and three pieces of bologna. Then, at night, she still had the ice cream snack but cut the portion in half.

	Calories
One slice baked ham (4″ × 4″)	50
One-half slice Swiss cheese (4″ × 4″)	65
One-half hard roll	78
Five ounces beer	63
One-quarter cup buttered noodles	60
Total	316

This example is a variation on the previous one, and shows how flexibility and experimentation will lead you to discover the most effective way for you to cut down your caloric overshoot without making yourself feel deprived. Walter does not feel satisfied unless the sandwich he is eating has a certain *thickness* to it, so he kept that the same, or even a bit bigger than before, except that now he is eating only *half* a sandwich.

But what's this business about 5 ounces of beer? No, I'm not going to ask you to pour the second half of that bottle of beer down the drain. Those 5 ounces of beer are what you don't drink if, instead of buying your beer in the usual 12-ounce bottle, you buy it by the pony, which contains only 7 ounces. True, not every brand comes in the pony size but there's precious little difference between one brand of beer and another anyway. At least American beer.

	Calories
One-half corn beef sandwich	175
One-third tablespoon salad oil	40
One Oreo cookie	50
One fig bar cookie	50
Total	315

The big deduction here comes from eliminating half of a corn beef sandwich, which for this person, is a typical Saturday night after-theater snack. What she did was convince her husband to split the sandwich with her rather than each ordering a whole one. They discovered that half a sandwich is quite enough to satisfy them. The reduction in the salad oil is gained by the simple expedient of tossing the salad more. And the two cookies represent the elimination of some "amusement" eating.

	Calories
One-half sausage link	35
One-half buttered pancake with syrup	90
Two saltines	24
One beer	151
Total	300

Here's another example of reducing by sharing. The husband and wife each typically had one sausage link and two pancakes for breakfast each day. Now, they cook only one link, and share it, and instead of grilling four pancakes, they make only three, sharing the third one. At dinner time, this person eats two saltines instead of the usual four, and has decided that she is going to cut out her nightly beer on Monday through Thursday evenings.

	Calories
One Coke	144
One-quarter cup creamed chipped beef	95
Two small chocolate-coated mints	90
Total	329

If you put all this food together, it wouldn't look like much, but when you overeat by this much every day, it does look like a lot when it builds up on your hips! That Coke could easily be replaced by water, club soda, or coffee. The small amount of creamed chipped beef is a second helping not taken, or perhaps a slightly smaller first helping. The two mints are typical examples of an "amusement" snack.

	Calories
One root beer	152
One piece of Boston brown bread with cream cheese	155
Total	307

Here is a good illustration of how a person who habitually eats a number of snack foods each day can accomplish the desired reduction by eliminating just two items. Two more "deuces" follow.

	Calories
Two cups buttered popcorn	82
Four graham crackers	220
Total	302

	Calories
One Twinkie	190
One cup Hawaiian Punch	110
Total	300

Three-quarters cup chocolate pudding 290 calories

And sometimes, as in this example and those below, the elimination of just *one* snack (which is eaten habitually) can achieve the desired reduction.

One piece marble cake 290 calories

One piece cherry pie 308 calories

One hot dog on a roll 295 calories

One Hostess fruit pie 460 calories

These single deductions seem to be letting the person off easy, but keep in mind that anyone who eats cake *every day* may be considerably overweight. In that case, it would be appropriate to increase the daily deductions, after about two months, to 400 calories a day.

Sometimes it's not a single item, but a single "assault" on a box or can or tray of snacks that can account for the sum of your daily caloric overshoot, and then some. For instance:

Six oatmeal raisin cookies	354 calories
Six fig bar cookies	300 calories
Two Ring Dings	320 calories

Sometimes the solution can be found in the elimination of one or two items, not ordinarily thought of as especially fattening, that are nibbled throughout the day. For instance:

		Calories
Fifteen very small cheese crackers		225
Five teaspoons sugar		75
	Total	300

In this example, the person typically drank about six cups of coffee a day. She found that she was able to learn to enjoy her coffee without sugar, except for the first cup of the day.

Some people who eat "health foods" almost exclusively find themselves overweight despite their avoidance of junk food. You can get some idea of why that may be so from looking at the next three examples:

		Calories
Three medium figs		120
One-half cup grape juice		83
Five large prunes		100
	Total	303

		Calories
Five dates		110
One-quarter cup dried peach halves		105
One tablespoon honey		64
Three unshelled peanuts		30
	Total	309

		Calories
Six walnuts		158
Six roasted almonds		46
Three Brazil nuts		93
	Total	297

As you can see at a glance, dried fruits and nuts (seeds, too) are not only nutritional gold mines, but caloric gold mines as well. It's one thing to eat them as part of the food you actually require — in fact, that's an excellent idea. But when you eat too much of these concentrated foods, the results quickly become obvious.

There are even some fresh fruits, popular among health food people, that pack a caloric wallop:

		Calories
One mango		152
One-half avocado		188
	Total	340

Notice the caloric density of just half an avocado, and keep it in mind the next time you think of making an avocado dip (guacamole).

While ordinarily you will be deducting foods eaten at a number of times throughout the day, it's quite possible that the elimination of just one snack time can turn the tide for you.

		Calories
One cherry soda		171
Six thin pretzels		140
	Total	311

Here's a teenager who, on returning from school each day, sits down in front of the TV and has a soda and a handful of pretzels. That may not sound like much, but it adds up. And sitting in front of the TV makes matters worse. In this case, the elimination of that one snack — which is accomplished by going out for 30 minutes of walking — was quite sufficient to achieve the desired weight loss and control.

Here's another example of a single snacking session, repeated on a daily basis, or close to it, that, if eliminated, would be sufficient to achieve a respectable weight loss:

	Calories
One 3½-ounce glass of white wine	87
One ounce cheddar cheese	113
Five rye wafers	100
Total	300

This example brings up an important point. *In deciding what you are not going to eat, it is vital to know what you can give up without feeling deprived and what you can't. To discover this may require repeated experimentation.*

For instance, in the example above, it's possible that the wine, cheese, and rye wafers don't represent merely so many calories, but a daily ritual which has come to be an important part of that person's life. It's something he looks forward to, something that helps him relax at the end of the workday. If he enjoys it with his wife, it may also be an important social or domestic event. If all that is the case, and the entire snack consists of what is listed above, you can imagine that simply whipping it out of the daily diet is going to create a troublesome vacuum. Of course, there are an infinite number of ways to fill that vacuum, including a shared walk, a shared hobby activity, or perhaps starting right in to make dinner together. *But that vacuum must be filled somehow.*

There's also the possibility that the food listed above consists of only *half* the wine and cheese consumed, and that halving the snack is not going to cause any feeling of deprivation.

Another possibility would be to modify the snack somewhat. For instance, along with the wine, each person might eat half an apple. Yet, even that slight change would deduct approximately 170 calories a day. The other 130 calories or so could be deducted elsewhere.

Of course, it's possible to defeat this kind of program by kidding yourself into believing that you ordinarily eat more than you really do. Let's say that you decide not to eat the following food on one particular day:

		Calories
One-half piece plain Danish		78
One-quarter cup bread pudding with raisins		125
One brownie with nuts		97
	Total	300

These deductions are only going to be meaningful if in fact you do habitually and typically eat at least this many calorie-rich snack items every day. If, in reality, you typically have one Coke, one serving of ice cream, and one brownie each day, and then decide to go on having the Coke and ice cream while cutting out the brownie, it isn't going to help to imagine that you're giving up a Danish and the bread pudding.

Self-examination is not the only quality needed to know where to cut the fat out of your diet. Flexibility is also important. During the week, for instance, you may find that removing 300 calories more or less from your daily diet involves not much more than giving up one can of soda and a cupcake. On Sunday, though, it can be a different story:

		Calories
One-quarter cup of stuffing		104
One-half tablespoon blue cheese dressing		40
One-quarter piece chocolate cake		90
One-half muffin		60
One-third pat butter		12
	Total	306

As you might have guessed, this entire reduction was cut out of one meal — Sunday dinner. And certainly, these deductions can be made from a big dinner without forcing you to go away from the table feeling hungry. Yet, they are perfectly valid as part of the program — *providing that you have typically been eating all these items or their equivalents every Sunday.*

Now, that may give you the idea that you could go a bit further with calorie-cutting on Sunday than you can during the week. And that might very well be true — so long as you don't go *too* far. You might, for instance, have half a pancake less for breakfast, and later in the evening, substitute club soda for your usual alcoholic beverage. If you *are* able to do that, it is perfectly permissible to feel that the extra couple of hundred calories you cut back on Sunday can be added back at some point during the week (a good time might be when you go out to a restaurant). Just be careful not to cut back *too much* on the weekends, because that could easily induce feelings of deprivation or even real hunger, either one of which could lead to a minor binge.

Another thing worth keeping in mind is that you should examine your diet very carefully for items which are relatively high in calories but which don't give you very much satisfaction. It wouldn't make much sense to cut out half a corn beef sandwich, which has about 175 calories, when you could cut out two macaroons and eliminate 180 calories — unless those two macaroons are going to bring you more satisfaction than half a sandwich. And if brownies bring you untold delight, you're better off allowing yourself half a brownie on any given day than cutting out that special treat while leaving in four saltines, which have just as many calories as half a brownie.

Since it's possible that cutting out 300 calories every day could be a bit difficult for you to handle, especially while you're still adjusting to the new eating patterns you'll be learning, it might be worthwhile to take a quick look at what 200 calories can look like:

	Calories
One-half bagel and cream cheese	110
One glass apricot nectar	107
Total	217

	Calories
One-half cup mashed potatoes (made with milk and butter)	99
One-half cup ice cream	127
Total	226

		Calories
Seven french fries		149
One-half glass dessert wine		70
	Total	219

		Calories
Five potato chips		55
One doughnut		164
	Total	219

		Calories
One tablespoon jelly		54
Two chocolate chip cookies		102
One slice salami		45
	Total	201

Finally, we should point out that it's quite possible to lose all the weight you want to without ever counting calories at all. After reading this book, and after paying more attention to your eating habits for a week or two, your consciousness of what you are eating will be raised to the point where you will probably be able to determine how much you are overeating, when, and why without recourse to any calorie charts. That knowledge will suggest ways in which that overeating can be eliminated.

But even if it serves no other purpose, the calculations that we've done here will bring into sharp focus several important points. They are that:

- Removing too many calories from the daily diet is worse — much worse — than not removing quite as many as you would like to. Removing fewer than you would like will only slow down your weight loss; removing too many is very likely to lead to feelings of deprivation which will in turn shake the foundations of your whole weight-loss program.
- A reasonable, realistic number of calories to cut out of the daily diet is 300. Many people will find that cutting out 200 or 250 is much easier to accomplish — which means that those people will get better results aiming for the lower daily deductions.

- It will not be difficult to find 300 calories that can be deducted from your daily diet without interfering with your nutritional needs or leading to hunger or feelings of deprivation. Snacks and second helpings should be your primary targets, not main dishes. As you lose weight, you can gradually increase the deductions, because your requirements will be significantly less.
- In selecting foods to be eliminated, make maximum use of self-knowledge, experimentation, and flexibility. Expect to have days that don't work out the way you had hoped; they will have no more effect on how long it takes you to reach your destination than hitting a red light does on a 100-mile drive. Just follow the map — you'll get there soon enough.

10

Undrink Yourself Thin

Usually, we think we're overweight because we eat too much. But in many cases, and perhaps in yours, that isn't the problem at all.

Our real downfall may be that we *drink* too much.

In fact, it is very likely that most people with a weight problem could completely overcome it and permanently control it without reducing by one ounce the amount of real food they eat. If they concentrated instead on changing what they *drink*, they'd be home free. If you think I'm exaggerating, consider these facts:

According to the most recent available statistics, the average American drinks in the course of one year:

- 1.8 gallons of liquor, containing nearly 7,000 calories;
- 2.7 gallons of wine, containing over 5,000 calories;
- 300 bottles of beer, containing 30,000 calories; and
- 67 gallons of soft drinks, containing approximately 46,000 calories.*

As incredible as it may seem, it's a fact that the average American consumes approximately 88,000 calories a year in the form of recreational beverages.

Even more shocking is the realization that those beverages are delivering the potential to create and maintain over 17 pounds of fat!

To better understand the implications of that fact, consider

* Approximately 12 percent of all soda consumed is diet soda. The caloric value has been adjusted to reflect this fact.

that all those calories contribute nothing to anyone's nutritional requirements. While it's true that beer has small amounts of the B-vitamin niacin, some potassium, and a dab of protein, and that table wine has some useful iron, the overall nutritional effect of alcoholic beverages is highly negative, because alcohol inhibits absorption of B vitamins, vitamin C, zinc, magnesium, and probably other nutrients as well.

So not only from the point of view of weight control, but because of some very serious health concerns, it's important for all of us to take a very close analytical look at our use of these recreational beverages.

One thing we do *not* want to do is to try to simply eliminate all these beverages from our diet. That kind of all-out assault on established eating and drinking patterns is totally alien to our new natural approach. The result could be a tremendous feeling of deprivation, which in turn would lead to disgust with the whole idea of weight control and eventually trigger a break-out binge of mindless indulgence. (Exactly *how* it's best to go about reducing the amount of calories we take in from recreational drinking we'll get to just a little bit later.)

The statistics we presented above are for the "average" person. It's easy, though, to get a good idea of how many calories *you* take in from these beverages — if you take the time to estimate *honestly* the quantity of these beverages you typically consume. Let's look at a few actual examples, from which you should be able to extrapolate the net effect that recreational drinking has on your own weight.

Robert said he never drinks beer, almost never touches wine, and although he does drink quite a bit of soda, he has always used diet soda. But he does drink scotch on the rocks, usually one a day, he said, each drink containing about 2 ounces of whiskey, which is a little bit more than the usual amount served in bars (1½ ounces). Each ounce of 86-proof scotch, like other whiskeys, contains 70 calories. Since each drink he consumes contains 2 ounces, that's 140 calories a day from liquor. Robert multiplied 140 calories by 365 days and was rather surprised (to put it mildly) that he was slurping down over 50,000 calories a year in his daily highballs. When consumed in addition to enough food to maintain weight, those calories can create and keep ten pounds of fat.

Eileen couldn't stand the taste of whiskey and, like Robert, drank only diet soda. But every day, with dinner, she drank two wine glasses of Chablis or sauterne. Such table wines contain 87 calories to the wine glass (3½ ounces), which meant that her daily two glasses of wine were providing 174 calories a day, 1,218 calories a week, and over 63,000 calories a year — enough to create and maintain 12 pounds of fat — just from a little wine.

Judy is a beer and soda drinker, habitually drinking one can of Coke a day, and about three bottles of beer a week, usually on weekends. One can of Coke has 144 calories, and a bottle of beer, 151, so Judy's weekly calories from beer and soda amounted to 1,461, or about 76,000 calories a year — resulting in an energy intake capable of producing 15 pounds of fat.

None of the participants in our workshop sessions were particularly heavy drinkers, or at least none considered themselves to be so. The heaviest drinker, though, was Hillary (like all the other participants, she isn't being identified by her real name). Hillary's case is extremely revealing, because she had been fighting a battle with her weight for many years and was not able to understand why it was so difficult for her to control (she was about 25 pounds too heavy) when she watched what she ate so closely. Hillary learned a lot about her weight-control problem when she conscientiously wrote down what she typically drank on a daily or weekly basis.

Every day, before dinner, she said, she and her husband spent half an hour over martinis, talking about what had happened to them on that particular day. Hillary herself usually sipped her way (quite enjoyably) through one double martini, which contained about three ounces of gin and a little bit of dry vermouth, for a total caloric punch of about 250 calories.

But in addition to the martinis, she said, she and her husband entertained or went to parties quite frequently, where she liked to have about two mixed drinks. She figured she had about four mixed drinks each week, containing a total of about 420 calories. That amounts to an average *daily* total of 310 calories. Hillary divided that by 14 and discovered that even if her food intake did not exceed her requirements, her drinking was enough to create and maintain 22 pounds of fat. Almost exactly the extent to which she was overweight.

A gold mine in reverse. You might want to think of your recreational beverage calories as a kind of gold mine in reverse: a rich lode of junk that will enrich your health and beautify your body as you dig it out and throw it away. But just like a real gold mine, this lode of empty calories must be treated with enormous respect for its structural integrity. If you attack it thoughtlessly, the whole thing is likely to come crashing down on your head: a catastrophic cave-in of motivation.

The key to successfully planning and executing the removal of a reasonable number of these junk drink calories from your daily diet is to determine very thoughtfully which of your drinking experiences bring you real pleasure and satisfaction and which do not. Once you do that, you will be in a position to apply certain tactical maneuvers which will carve out and neatly dispose of a substantial number of unneeded calories. Exactly how many calories you eliminate depends entirely on your own drinking habits and values, as we will soon discover.

Let's begin the "action" part of this chapter by considering which drinks we take really mean something to us, and *what* they mean.

We discovered in our workshop sessions that although many people habitually drank soda, only a few said they found it a very enjoyable or meaningful experience. One person always had Coke with lunch because it seemed to go well with hamburgers and french fries. It wasn't so much that the Coke was enjoyable, but that the thought of drinking water with french fries seemed almost bizarre. For health reasons, we do not suggest drinking diet soda, even though we've observed that some people wean themselves off soda altogether after drinking diet soda for a while. So, we suggested to Paula that if she were going to continue to eat a portion of french fries with her hamburger, she should eat the french fries first, and then the hamburger. After the hamburger, she could have a cup of coffee, which *did* seem to blend well with the lingering taste of the hamburger. Although coffee is certainly not a health drink, a cup of coffee, even with sugar and milk in it, still has about 100 calories less than a can of Coke. Coke, of course, has a significant amount of caffeine in it anyway, and the enormous amount of sugar it contains probably does more harm to your metabolism than the caffeine in coffee.

Theresa also drank Coke every day, during her afternoon break. There was no Coke machine where she worked, so she would bring a can with her and keep it in the refrigerator in the snack area. "At first, I thought I really needed that Coke every day; that's why I brought it with me. I thought I would get really tired and sleepy without it. But one of the first things I did on the weight-control program was to try leaving the Coke at home and drinking water instead. After taking a long drink from the water fountain, I would walk around the building for about five minutes so I wouldn't have to watch the other women drinking soda and coffee. I was amazed to discover that I hardly missed the Coke at all, and after about a week, I had no desire for soda anymore. Whatever the Coke was doing for me, taking a drink of water and going for a quick walk was just as good."

To help her accomplish this reduction of 144 calories a day from a junk drink, Theresa was using autosuggestion every evening, a very simple and very natural process which we'll describe later. She was telling herself: *"When I drink water, I'm choosing to become slender. Drinking water is like washing my fat away."*

Some people appear to be actually addicted to Coke. They seem to require the "rush" produced by the sugar and caffeine, sometimes drinking Coke and coffee throughout the day to try to keep up their energy. But drinking Coke and an excessive amount of coffee only aggravates energy "brownouts." In some cases, these junk drinks are fueling the fires of reactive hypoglycemia — blood glucose levels that bounce violently up and down under the influence of sugar. Other people who swig Coke and coffee frequently through the day do so largely out of habit and for the sake of putting something into their mouths. The best course of action here is to immediately begin cutting down on soda drinking and substituting water. It should not take more than a week or two until you feel quite comfortable without these drinks. In fact, you'll probably feel great, as your energy levels will be steadier and your ego will glow with the realization that you've eliminated all those needless empty calories so easily.

Other people drink soda without even thinking about it. When their throat feels a little dry, they open the refrigerator and there's the bottle of orange soda. Or they use soda to wash down their food during meals. That kind of junk drink consumption is the easiest to eliminate. If you have to have soda in your house because other family members demand it, remind yourself that drinking soda is like drinking pure fat; drinking water is like washing away your weight problem.

Reducing your consumption of alcoholic beverages is somewhat more challenging. In fact, you may find the process quite fascinating and educational, because you will learn a lot about human behavior in the process.

The first step is to have a very clear picture in your mind of your drinking behavior. It helps a lot to spend about ten minutes with paper and pencil and write down your observations, adding to the information and revising it as you continue your analysis.

Before even thinking about how much you drink, think about *when* you drink. And *where* you drink. Keep in mind that you aren't judging yourself — there are no moral issues here. All you want to do is analyze an important part of your dietary behavior.

Do you sip wine while doing housework? Do you have a cocktail during lunch at a restaurant? Every day? Just on Friday? Do you open a bottle of beer immediately after coming home from work? Do you drink it while reading the newspaper? Or while talking with your spouse? Do you drink later in the evening while watching TV? Do you drink before going to bed? Do you drink before having dinner at a restaurant? When friends come over to your house to visit? When you visit friends at their house? Parties? Business functions?

At this point, you may be beginning to realize that drinking alcoholic beverages is a habit which has been socially sanctioned at almost every conceivable kind of function and activity. Keep thinking. Do you drink beer at ball games? Do you have a cocktail in the clubhouse after playing golf? Do you go out for beers after playing tennis? Do you drink in the theater lobby between acts of a play or opera? Do you drink after religious services? At wakes or at funeral-related rituals? At weddings? Baptisms? Bar mitzvahs? Lodge meetings? Do you take a six-pack of beer with you when you go fishing? Do you carry along wine when you go on a picnic? In warm weather, do you drink gin and tonics to cool off? Do you like to have a hot toddy to warm up?

Curious, isn't it, how often and at how many different places contemporary standards permit — actually *encourage* — drinking. Such social conventions lead many people to behave like alcoholics even though they aren't. Alcoholism aside — it's simply beyond the scope of this book — there is no doubt that our modern drinking customs go a long way towards encouraging us to slurp down an astonishing number of calories.

Now that you have a pretty clear idea of when and where you drink (again, it's a good idea to write your individual pattern down so you can literally see it), the next step is to go over the list and note *how much* you typically drink under each of these various circumstances. There are two important reasons for doing this. First, you will be giving yourself an accounting of the approximate number of calories you're habitually taking in from alcoholic beverages. Second, and actually more important, an accounting will be of great help to you in deciding where it will be most productive to modify your drinking behavior.

Warren made a list that looked like this:

one business lunch per week = 2 drinks/week
at hotels when traveling = 2 drinks/week
at parties, etc., about once a month = ½ drink/week
at hockey games, about 12 a year (2 beers per game) = ½ beer/week
after golf, about 15 times a year, 2 beers each time = ½ beer/week
after mowing lawn, about 24 times a year = ½ beer/week
at night to feel sleepy, about once a week = 1 beer/week

Once a year, Warren went to a business convention where he drank "incredible" amounts of liquor and beer, but since he only did this on one weekend a year, he omitted it from his list, which is perfectly all right.

Calculating that one drink of liquor is equal to about 105 calories, while one beer equals 150 calories, Warren's accounting revealed that on a weekly basis, he was consuming about 475 calories from liquor and 375 calories from beer, or an average daily total of 121 calories from alcohol. Dividing by 14, he discovered that alcohol was providing him with enough calories to create and "nourish" more than eight pounds of fat.

At this point, if you haven't done so already, you should give yourself the benefit of an accounting of both when and approximately how much you typically drink.

Now that you have a pretty clear idea of when, where, and how much you drink, it's time to begin thinking about a question that's even more fun to play with. Namely, *why* do you drink at those times and places?

We spent about 15 minutes with Warren reviewing this question and here is what he said:

About once a week, he takes a client out to lunch and usually has a drink before eating and another after. He does this, he said, for two reasons. First, because the drink before eating makes him relax, and second, because he feels it would be impolite not to encourage the client to drink (a good example of our contemporary drinking customs at work). Usually, he added, he had no particular desire for a glass of port or a brandy after lunch, but he thought it was good for business to share that extra drink with the client.

Warren was on the road an average of one day a week, and he said it was "comforting" to have a drink with dinner and another before going to bed, to help him sleep.

At the parties and functions which he attended on the average of once a month, he said he usually had two drinks "because it's fun to drink at parties." It is also "fun," he said, to have a couple of beers at hockey games and after playing golf.

After mowing the lawn he liked to have a beer because he felt so thirsty, and because it was a kind of reward for an hour of cutting grass in the hot sun.

Finally, about once a week he had a beer late at night when he felt he was not sleepy but ought to go to bed. The beer helped him sleep, he said.

Hillary, whom we mentioned before, essentially drank in only two situations: before dinner every night, when she enjoyed a 250-calorie double martini, and while entertaining or attending parties, which she did frequently.

Hillary said that the nightly cocktail with her husband was a kind of ritual she looked forward to. She and her husband relaxed, talked about what had happened to them during the day, and in general seemed to reinforce their ties. And why did she drink at parties? "Well, when someone comes over to your house, you have to be a gracious host or hostess, and when you go over to someone else's house, well, they're always putting a drink in your hands. And after you have a couple of drinks, you seem to be having a better time."

These two examples give us some idea of the surprisingly wide range of reasons that people drink. Business etiquette, loneliness, a desire to fall asleep faster, family rituals, fun and games, and sheer physical thirst are only a few.

In deciding where to begin changing your drinking behavior, *experiment aggressively with changing drinking behavior which seems to be a result of habit, a desire to be "doing something," or a simple need to satisfy thirst.*

The second principle is: *in those situations which are heavily ritualized or charged with emotional meaning, and which involve having more than one drink, experiment with reducing the amount consumed without destroying the social or emotional meaning.*

In Warren's case, the bulk of his alcohol calories were coming from liquor which he drank in situations associated with his business life. That fact in itself in no way means that Warren ought to devote all his energy to reducing those particular calories, but it was, at least, a place to begin.

"How do you feel about the fact," I asked him, "that someone is expected to abuse his body and his health because of his job?"

Warren thought for a moment and came up with an answer that caught me by surprise. "Hockey players do it all the time," he said. "So do firemen . . . garbage collectors. Even tennis players ruin their elbows and knees."

Since Warren obviously believed that there was nothing morally or ethically wrong about drinking in the expectation that it would help his job performance, I decided there was no benefit to be gained by attempting to convince him otherwise. Whether or not his belief was reasonable was entirely beside the point.

"Having one drink before a business lunch is very common. Having a drink after lunch is not exactly required behavior, is it?"

"No, I guess not."

"What do you say to the client before ordering that second drink?"

"Oh, I'll say 'How about a glass of port or a brandy?'"

"Suppose you said something like this: *'That was a good lunch. Do you feel like having another drink?'* Do you think that would be acceptable?"

"Yes, I could say that."

"And what do you think would happen?"

"Probably, the person would say 'No thanks' at least half the time."

"Then it's worth trying, because that would save you over 5,000 calories a year. You'd still have the opportunity to talk business over coffee, and your energy level during the rest of the afternoon would be much smoother."

Now, you might think that saving 100 calories a week is trivial, but it isn't — and not only because it adds up to over 5,000 calories a year. Any time you are able to modify your habitual behavior for the sake of your total well-being, you prove to yourself that you're in charge of your behavior and not the other way around. Every success helps build confidence.

I purposely did not get involved with questioning Warren's drinking behavior while on the road. Staying in hotels by yourself on business trips is boring, lonely, and for some people, emotionally stressful. In the early stages of the program, I did not feel that it was a good idea to "threaten" Warren with taking away his out-of-town drinking — which he was clearly using as a tranquilizer.

"When you attend hockey games, do you think it would spoil your fun if instead of having two beers you had only one?"

"Probably not. . . . I could try it, anyway, and see."

"And after playing golf, when you also have a couple of beers, do you drink more or less by yourself, or with a group of friends and make a kind of ritual out of it?"

"Sometimes by myself; sometimes with friends."

"And again, how do you think it would be if in the locker room, you drank a glass or two of water from the fountain and then only had one beer in the clubhouse?"

"That sounds like a good idea."

"After mowing the lawn, you say, you like to sit down with a beer. Well, after mowing the lawn, of course, you're very thirsty. Maybe that's most of the reason why you enjoy that beer so much. Do you think so?"

"Well, sure, I'm thirsty — but drinking beer is more fun than drinking water."

"Why don't you just try it once or twice, and tell yourself when you're pouring that glass of water, 'This water is going to wash away my fat.'"

"I guess I could try it."

Hillary's drinking revolved around two different situations, both of them involving social rituals: before-dinner cocktails with her husband, and drinks at the parties she enjoyed attending so much.

The first thing I asked her was if she was actually *thirsty* when she and her husband sat down to have their martinis. She replied that she wasn't certain. I suggested that immediately upon returning home she should try drinking a long, cool glass of water. If her alcohol drinking was prompted even in part by real thirst (which is often the case) she might find it quite acceptable to gradually reduce the amount of gin in her drink to just one jigger instead of two. That simple change could lop off seven pounds.

It's important to realize that when a person habitually sits down to two or more drinks at a certain time of the day, he is chemically tranquilizing himself. In some cases, there is no special need for tranquilization or even relaxation; the drinking is only a kind of social ritual. When two people drink together, one may need tranquilization while the other keeps up drink for drink as a gesture of friendliness. In such cases, both people may be able to break out of this fattening habit rather easily, simply by *making plans* to do something else *together* — whether it be taking a walk, preparing dinner, working on the garden or shrubbery, or maybe even showering together or making love.

Hillary seemed to be rather high-strung, and I imagined that she did in fact require some relaxation. But drinking to relax — *on a daily basis* — is simply not a very good idea. It is fattening, addictive, and not at all conducive to developing the kind of relaxation that makes you feel better all through the day and gives you more restful sleep at night.

If you, like Hillary, drink for relaxation, you should realize that the important question is not really how little liquor you can drink and still get the desired effect, but *what you can do other than drinking to unwind.*

If there is a social ritual involved, as there was in Hillary's case, that ritual can be changed from one that is essentially narcotic in nature to one which is truly social or interpersonal, in the sense that what you are enjoying, and what makes you feel relaxed and secure, is the *other person's company.*

There are many ways to go about doing that. I suggested several of them to Hillary and urged her to try one or more. She might, for instance, try taking a 30-minute walk with her husband as soon as they both return from their jobs. That would be at least as relaxing as a jigger of gin, and would burn up 150 calories instead of adding 100 calories. When they return from the walk, they could still have their drinks, but they would in all likelihood find that one drink instead of two was quite enough to bring them to the desired state of mellowness.

Some people find that listening to their favorite music for about 15 minutes is all it takes to unwind them after a day's work. Records are far better for this purpose than radio. And listening to the music gives you the required "backdrop" for the ritual, lessening your dependence on alcohol.

I'd suggest trying any one or more of these approaches. Just remember one thing: *plan ahead for what you are going to do during these daily rituals.* If you wait until the time for them is upon you, you will more than likely let the momentum of habit sweep you into a repetition of the same old pattern.

Warren went to parties only about once a month, where he

had about two drinks, which I did not think was worth very much attention. Hillary, however, drinks in social situations on the average of twice a week — which *does* merit some attention. And in fact, it didn't take Hillary long to cut her drinking in half in these situations. "All I really wanted," she told us, "was that first drink. After that, I was drinking just to be polite. So now, what I do is have the first drink, and then after that fill my glass with club soda. Everyone else figures I'm drinking, so they don't bother me. What I also do, when possible, is go into another room, where there are no bottles of liquor or snacks and do my talking there. I have just as good a time doing that, and it makes me feel good when I leave because I don't feel guilty about having done something that I really didn't want to do."

I don't recommend drinking club soda as a regular beverage because of its acidity, but at parties, if you make your second and third drinks club soda with a twist of lime, you can sip away with everyone else while washing away your fat. Ginger ale is a compromise:two small glasses have the same number of calories as one shot of liquor.

When *you* are the host at a party or get-together, you might want to announce that besides the usual drinks, you have Perrier or some other brand of sparkling water. After one drink of liquor, you may find that many of the guests will enjoy drinking this sparkling water with a slice of lime. It is a much more pleasant drink than club soda and contains no chemicals of any kind, being naturally carbonated. If you can afford it, it's a great idea to have a bottle of sparkling spring water in the refrigerator at all times. Although it may seem expensive compared to tap water, or even some bottled waters, these imported sparkling waters cost about half as much as very inexpensive wine. So if you are accustomed to sipping wine, you will do yourself a big favor by drinking sparkling water instead, and it won't cost you a penny more.

Most of us don't usually think of our coffee- or tea-drinking habits as contributing significantly to our weight problems, but we may be overlooking a valuable vein in the gold mine of junk calories presented by recreational beverages.

While coffee and tea in and of themselves do not contain a significant number of calories, the way we serve them is another story. Sylvia, for example, drank five cups of coffee a day — with one level teaspoon of sugar in each cup. That meant a total of 75 calories a day from sugar in her coffee — an astonishing total of over 27,000 calories a year.

But besides adding sugar to her coffee, she also added milk — about two tablespoons to each cup. At about 10 calories per tablespoon, that meant another 36,000 calories. So just in drinking her five daily cups of coffee, Sylvia was ingesting enough calories to subsidize nine extra pounds.

I never suggest to people that they quit putting milk in their coffee, because most people can use the calcium it contains, and milk tends to counteract some of the bad effects that both coffee and tea have on our bodies. But sugar is a different story. I suggested that Sylvia try what had worked for a friend of mine. One day, pretty much by accident, he sat down to have a cup of coffee which he had forgotten to sweeten with sugar. Feeling too lazy to get up and get sugar, he drank it the way it was and discovered to his surprise that it wasn't all that bad. By the next day, he was drinking all his coffee without sugar, except for his first cup in the morning.

If you lighten your coffee with something other than milk, consider that while milk has about 10 calories to a tablespoon, half-and-half has 20, light cream has 32, light cream for whipping has 45, and heavy cream 55.

While there is usually a limit to how much milk or cream you can put into coffee, some people drink what I've heard referred to as New England tea, which consists of one-half strong tea and one-half milk, sometimes with cream added. After brewing the strong tea, you add the milk or cream, a relatively large amount of sugar, heat and serve. That kind of brew has over 100 calories a cup.

But it literally isn't half as bad as a cup of cocoa made with milk, which delivers about 230 calories. If you like to have a cup of cocoa before retiring, I suggest you try hot milk instead, which will give you only 80 calories — and a better night's sleep to boot, because while cocoa contains theobromine, a stimulant, milk contains the amino acid tryptophan, a natural tranquilizer.

A surprising number of people I've met abuse still another beverage — fruit juice. Usually, these people have been turned on to health food, and the first thing they do is quit drinking soda pop. They replace it with fruit juice which they commence to drink like water, never thinking that natural sugars are much more concentrated in fruit juices than they are in raw fruits. One cup of grape juice, for instance, has 167 calories — more calories than you would get by eating 80 of the grapes that juice was made from!

Eric said that after changing over to a health food kind of a diet, he was drinking about a quart of orange juice a day. "Every time I was thirsty, I would have another glass of orange juice. Now I have one glass a day, and drink water the rest of the time."

Eric made another change in his drinking behavior which also saved him a lot of calories. "I used to drink several cups of herb tea every day, which I would sweeten with honey. I stopped using the honey and switched to mint and chamomile tea, which tastes good without any sweetener." Personally, I don't like chamomile tea without some kind of sweetener, so when I drink it, I add a slug of orange juice. But most people will find that it won't take them long to learn to enjoy peppermint or spearmint tea "straight."

11

How Natural Foods Can Help You Lose Weight

One of the most basic and healthful strategies you can apply in your weight-control program is to emphasize natural foods in your daily diet.

Notice I said "emphasize." I didn't say you have to (or even should) eat *only* natural foods. Nor did I say you have to eat unusual foods, or shop only in health food stores. You can buy 80 to 90 percent of the natural foods you will need to hasten and help maintain your weight loss in any first-class supermarket.

Why should you emphasize natural foods? The answer to that one is easy: *Natural foods are much less fattening than processed or convenience foods.* There are exceptions, of course, but that's the general rule. Looking at it another way, natural foods are to be preferred because you can better satisfy your appetite by eating relatively larger amounts of them than you can by eating smaller amounts of high-calorie convenience foods.

What's more, we aren't talking about a marginal difference of 40 or 50 calories a day, but of 100, 200, or even more calories a day — and that's just from *emphasizing* natural foods, not eating them exclusively.

But just what *are* natural foods, anyway? That can be a mighty difficult and tricky question to answer if you try to frame your answer in highly technical or absolute terms. Many typewriter ribbons have been pounded into lace (no one spills ink anymore) trying to do just that. And all for naught. People don't seem to realize that "natural" is a *relative* word. Foods are natural by degree, not in an absolute yes-or-no sense. And while nearly all foods are natural to some extent, some foods are more natural than others.

To determine the relative degree to which a food is natural, all you have to do is ask yourself how close it is to the state in which it came from nature. The greater the number of additions, of subtractions, and of modifications, the less natural it is.

And about nine times out of ten, these changes involve:

- the addition of sugar or other sweeteners;
- the addition of fats or oils; and
- the removal of fiber.

Of course, there are other characteristic changes as well, most notably the loss of vitamins and minerals; the degradation of taste; the addition of preservatives, artificial coloring agents, and other chemicals; and the addition of salt (which can lead to retention of water and even high blood pressure). But purely from the perspective of weight control, the critical changes which occur in food processing are the addition of sugar, the addition of fat, and the removal of fiber or natural bulk. The net results of these changes, needless to say, are unwanted and entirely unnecessary calories.

Let's get down to some specifics.

The potato is a perfect example of what happens to a basically honest and nourishing food when food processors get hold of it. Probably the most natural way you can prepare a potato is simply to bake it in its skin. Do that and you have something which is quite filling, yet contains only 145 calories (less than two slices of white bread, and that's for a large potato). You get good vitamins too, including 20 milligrams of vitamin C. As for fat, there's so little in a baked potato that analysis can discover only a trace.

Now, if you were to eat french fries instead of a baked potato, you would probably eat about ten fries (each four inches long). But instead of getting 145 calories, you'd get 214 — an increase of 47 percent. And instead of getting 30 milligrams of vitamin C, you'd get only 16, a *decrease* of 47 percent.

Now, let's say that instead of french fries, you were going to eat potato chips, but since they're taking the place of the french fries or the baked potato, you have to eat enough to satisfy your appetite. It's hard to say exactly how many potato chips that might be, but I'd estimate that if you were eating small chips, each only about two inches in diameter, you would wind up eating around 20 before you reached the same sensation of fullness or satisfaction you'd get from one baked potato.

But when you eat those 20 small chips, you're getting 228 calories, about 50 percent more than you get from the baked potato and a little more than from the french fries. And as for the vitamin C, you get only a miserable six milligrams.

But that isn't the end of the story. Foods are not consumed in a vacuum, and we shouldn't look at them with the same narrow perspective that a scientist might use. Let's use the holistic approach. In this case, ask yourself what you're going to *drink* after you eat your potatoes. Eating a baked potato doesn't make you particularly thirsty, because 75 percent of it actually *is* water. French fries, however, are only 45 percent water, and potato chips just 2 percent water. Even more important, both french fries and potato chips are likely to be loaded with salt, which makes you thirsty. And when you're eating french fries or potato chips, what is it you feel like drinking to slake your thirst? Water? Not very likely. Chances are, you're going to drink soda or beer, adding empty calories from sugar to the empty calories from all the fat in the potato chips.

To be fair, we should probably assume that you're going to eat that baked potato with a pat of butter. But even with the butter, your total calories will only be about 180, and your total fat about half of that in the french fries, and just one-quarter of the amount in the potato chips.

This little bit of nutritional accountancy has several morals, but one of them is *not* that you should *never* eat french fries or potato chips again as long as you live. Rather, as often as you feel like it, you should *plan* on having a baked potato instead of french fries or chips. Or eat a potato boiled in its skin, which is also virtually fat-free and perfectly nutritious. Every time you do that, you'll save from 40 to 60 calories.

Fresh fruit versus canned fruit is another good example of the effect of food processing on calories. If you eat a peach for dessert, you get something sweet and tasty that has about 60 calories. If you eat a peach that was canned in heavy syrup, you get something that's *very* sweet, not all that tasty, and has 126 calories — a caloric increase of more than 100 percent. And that, mind you, is the smallest canned peach on the market. If you eat one of the largest kind, you'd get 170 calories!

Do you enjoy the taste of fresh blueberries? If you were to indulge yourself when they're in season by eating a whole cupful, you would be getting 90 calories. But eat the same cupful of blueberries canned and sweetened — a kind frequently sold in supermarkets — and instead of 90 calories, you're getting 229.

Do you like fresh sweet cherries? Eat a whole cup of fresh cherries and you've just taken in 82 calories — not all that bad for a delicious snack that's only available for a few weeks a year. But if you eat your cherries canned in syrup, that same cupful is going to sock you with almost 210 calories.

In fact, you'd be better off eating a whole cup of fresh cherries than eating just half a cup of canned cherries — that's how many extra calories are added by the syrup.

If instead of eating that cup of canned cherries, you were to have a small piece of cherry pie, the calories would climb all the way up to about 310. Choosing the pie instead of the cup of fresh cherries costs you 230 calories. At that price, don't you think you could learn to enjoy fresh, *natural* food as much as the cooked, sugar-laden pie? (To exercise away the difference between the two, you'd have to walk about two miles!)

With apple pie, it's the same story. One small piece of the pie has almost as many calories as four whole apples. Enjoy one good-size apple instead of a piece of pie and you've done as much for your waistline as you would by walking rapidly for three-quarters of an hour.

For breakfast, I often enjoy a whole grapefruit cut into wedges, which has about 80 calories. If instead of the fresh fruit, I ate one cup of sweetened grapefruit sections from a can, I'd be slipping myself an *extra* 100 calories.

Of course, it's possible to eat canned fruit packed in water instead of syrup. If you do that, the vitamins may be significantly reduced, but the calories aren't all that different from fresh fruit. But I'd urge you to try to get into the habit of eating the fresh fruit instead of the water-packed canned variety, because the missing vitamins are important, and the taste of the fresh fruit is much better. Canned fruit packed in water is really blah.

You may be surprised to discover — as I was — that a slice of white bread weighing exactly the same as a slice of whole wheat bread has about 10 more calories than the more natural product — about 75 versus 65. That doesn't sound like a great deal, but if you eat two pieces of bread a day, the difference adds up to about 7,000 calories a year.

How fiber fights fat. Far more important though, than the caloric difference, is the big difference in fiber content between white bread and whole wheat bread. Portions of the wheat germ and bran which remain in the whole wheat product give it a total of eight times more fiber than white bread. That's important for many reasons, but to a person watching his weight, what it means is that whole wheat bread is going to be chewier, take longer to eat, be more filling, and in general, slow down your eating machine. The same goes for the fiber in fresh vegetables, fruits, potatoes, beans, and other natural foods, which are sometimes referred to as "complex carbohydrates."

Most of us probably know that foods with a lot of fiber take longer to eat and fill us up more. But how many, I wonder, realize that *including fibrous foods in your diet actually reduces the extent to which you can absorb calories from your food.* That most interesting fact was revealed in a study carried out jointly by the United States Department of Agriculture and the University of Maryland, and reported in 1978. A dozen adult men were put on a low-fiber diet for 26 days, and a high-fiber diet for another 26 days. Although their change in body weight, if any, was not reported, careful analysis revealed that on the high-fiber diet, there was a 4.8 percent decrease of calorie digestibility compared to the low-fiber diet. That's a significant percentage, amounting to 86 fewer calories a day absorbed on a diet consisting of 1,800 calories, and 120 fewer calories a day absorbed from a diet of 2,500 calories.

Some people might object that this is not a fair comparison, because the low-fiber diet might have been unnatural. But I don't think it was all that unusual. A typical low-fiber breakfast consisted of grapefruit juice, puffed rice, milk, an egg, toast with butter and jelly, and coffee with cream and sugar. A typical lunch was a tuna fish sandwich with mayonnaise on white bread and a glass of apple juice. A typical dinner included vegetable juice, ground beef and macaroni, a white roll, grape juice, and ice cream. Sounds pretty typical to me, although most people would have a piece of fresh fruit at least once in a while.

If the low-fiber diet wasn't all that different from what many people eat, neither was the high-fiber diet. In fact, I wouldn't even call it a "high-fiber" diet; it's just *relatively* higher. The only items in a day's worth of eating on the high-fiber diet that did in fact include any fiber were grapefruit, puffed rice, a serving of dates, three pieces of white bread, a serving of corn, some pineapple tidbits, one serving each of spinach, carrots, and cabbage, and blackberries for dessert.

In fact, the authors of the study — June L. Kelsay, Ph. D. and colleagues — purposely designed the high-fiber diet so it wouldn't include any whole-grain products. Her idea, I suppose, was to see if a moderate amount of fruit and vegetables would make a difference in the excretion of calories and other nutrients. And of course, it did. While 96.3 percent of the calories consumed in the low-fiber diet were absorbed, only 91.6 percent of those in the high-fiber diet actually passed through the intestinal tract and into the system where they could provide energy — and fat power.

It seems to me, although I have no data to prove it, that if you put some *real* fiber in your diet, you would get a substantially greater decrease in absorbed calories. And in fact, I suggest that you do just that. *Gradually.* Why go on eating white bread, when whole wheat bread not only tastes better, and contains fewer calories to begin with, but has so much more fiber? Do you *always* have to eat mushy stuff like puffed rice or eggs for breakfast? Why not try some hot oatmeal, with a teaspoon or two of bran mixed into it? Or some sugarless granola? As for lunch and dinner, I'd suggest that you make good friends with potatoes, beans, peas, soybeans, brown rice, carrots, cabbage, and turnips. If you have any taste at all for slightly exotic grains, try millet, barley, or buckwheat. You'll find plenty of excellent recipes for these kinds of foods in any good natural foods cookbook. Change your diet slowly, and don't continue eating anything you don't develop a taste for after eating it several times.

Focusing on these kinds of high-fiber foods will give you even more bonuses than a greater sensation of being filled and a reduction of calorie digestibility. High-fiber foods also tend to lower circulating levels of insulin, a hormone which is believed to stimulate appetite. They probably do that simply by making you *need* less insulin. One theory is that with all that fiber, your food is digested much more slowly, and sugar is entering your system at a slow, steady pace, instead of in one big burst. Another important bonus is that a high-fiber diet may tend to lower elevated blood pressure. In the study by Kelsay and colleagues, 6 out of the 12 men had a diastolic blood pressure averaging 88 while they were on the low-fiber diet (80 is normal). On the high-fiber diet, the average diastolic blood pressure dropped to 78.

That difference could be extremely significant, because diastolic blood pressure is not lowered all that readily, and is considered to be much more important than systolic blood pressure, which is the higher of the two numbers that make up your blood pressure portrait. Actually, the systolic blood pressure also fell in the study, but not to the extent of the diastolic.

Now, I don't want to exaggerate the importance of fiber to the weight reducer, because the truth is that fiber or bulk is not the only thing that signals your system that you're "full." Research indicates that the fat and protein content of the meal are also very important. In fact, it's perfectly possible to eat an enormous salad and still not really feel satisfied, because you haven't given your system any appreciable amount of protein or fat. Just the same, fiber is another factor in giving you that satisfied feeling. And it isn't just the fiber in natural foods that help fill you up, but their water content and crispness. Canned peaches, for instance, slip down the throat much more easily than raw peaches; eating three canned peach halves is no great challenge, but eating three raw peaches is.

Some foods which are usually thought of as natural really aren't all that natural (remember, natural is a relative word). In fact, two foods that have become the very symbols of "natural food" in the commercial marketplace have in truth been subjected to some "classic" food processing. I'm talking about granola and yogurt.

Granola. Take a good, close look at the ingredients label on some granola boxes — either in a supermarket or health food store. The first ingredient listed may be oats, which means that there are more oats in the granola than any other single ingredient. But keep going. The second ingredient is probably brown sugar. Then, a few items down, you'll come to honey. What's happening here is that the manufacturer has divided his sweetening agent into two different sources so that he can avoid having brown sugar as the largest single ingredient. Some manufacturers have three or four different sweeteners in their granolas: brown sugar, honey, corn sweetener, date sugar or dried dates, and raisins can all be used to add sugar in one form or another (dried fruits like dates and raisins are loaded with natural sugars) without being forced by labeling laws to list sugar as the first ingredient.

Keep studying that granola label. Among the first few ingredients, you'll also probably find "vegetable oil," which might very well be coconut oil, one of the few vegetable oils containing saturated fat. What I really find objectionable about the oil added to granola is that many of the key ingredients in granola are already *naturally* rich in oil: all kinds of nuts and seeds and even wheat.

The net result of these additions is a product that . . . well, just look at that label again. How many calories to the ounce? Probably, somewhere between about 110 and 125. Some manufacturers list one ounce as "one serving," but while that may be true for a small child, in my experience the typical adult is going to eat at least two ounces at a time. Add another 80 calories for half a cup of milk and you're talking about 300 calories or so for a serving of granola. Not that there's anything wrong with a 300-calorie breakfast — but once more, go back to that label and see how much protein and vitamin value you're getting for those 300 calories. The answer will vary depending on the formula (some granola makers fortify their products with dried milk or yeast), but in general, between the cereal *and* the milk, you're lucky to get about 10 grams of protein (half of which comes from the milk, not the granola). For the same number of calories — about 300 — you could have two scrambled eggs and a piece of lightly buttered whole wheat toast and get 17 grams of protein — 70 percent more protein for your caloric money.

But what I personally find much more objectionable about commercial granola as a food for the weight-conscious person is that it can be eaten like candy right out of the box. And many people do just that. In fact, it's even too easy to take second and third helpings of granola with milk. I can't remember ever eating a couple of eggs and a piece of toast and then going back and cooking a second helping, but I can remember all too well demolishing one-third or more of a box of granola at one sitting. And although I've experimented with making my own granola, using as little oil and honey as possible and fortifying it heavily with brewer's yeast, I find that I'm still unable to control my intake of this delicious "natural candy." So I've been forced to exclude it completely from my diet. If I want cereal in the morning, I have a hot bowl of oatmeal that I prepare with a lot of milk. I find it much more satisfying than the granola and I never even think about making a second bowl.

I'm not suggesting that everyone has to exclude granola from their pantry, though. If you can control your intake, I'd suggest you prepare your own, going as easy as possible on oils, sugars, and nuts, and fortifying it with dried skim milk, brewer's yeast, and fresh fruit.

Try to work some wheat germ and bran into the formula, too. But if you aren't going to make your own granola, think twice about having it around the house.

Yogurt. Just now I've gone to my refrigerator and taken out a familiar eight-ounce carton of yogurt. Looking at the labeling, I see that the contents have 150 calories. Do you have a carton of yogurt in your refrigerator? If you do, take a look at it and see what the calorie count is. If it's a flavored yogurt, like blueberry or strawberry, it probably has about 260 or 280 calories. Why the big difference? Simple. The kind of yogurt I've been eating lately is "plain." Don't be confused by the "low fat" legend that most yogurts have. The important story about yogurt is not fat, but sugar. Yes, plain, ordinary sugar. The small amount of fruit that's in a carton of flavored yogurt contains possibly 30 calories — which means that the rest of the extra calories — 100 of the little buggers — are all from the sugar in the fruit syrup.

In other words, if you figure that a teaspoon of sugar has 15 calories (which we are in this book, in keeping with the values given in government publications) your fruit-flavored yogurt contains the equivalent of six teaspoons of table sugar — and you say you thought yogurt was a *health* food?

Sure, yogurt is a health food — when it's really yogurt. When I recently traveled through the Caucasus region of the Soviet Union, I had yogurt or a form of it they call *kefir* almost everywhere I went. It's of a looser consistency than our yogurt, and is served cold in a cup with a sprig of mint. You drink it down and it tastes pretty much like buttermilk. The calorie content of that kind of yogurt will vary with the fat content of the milk, but it will be somewhere between 115 and 160 per cup. If you make your own yogurt at home from whole milk, it will have about 160 calories — the same number of calories as a cup of milk. Commercial yogurt is often made from partially skimmed milk, often mixed with milk solids, so again, the calorie count can vary somewhat. But it probably won't go over about 160.

In some supermarkets I have been in, they don't have any real yogurt at all. What they have is a chemicalized dessert concoction which contains artificial flavoring and coloring, starch to provide consistency, preservatives, and either lots of sugar or artificial sweeteners. And the beneficial yogurt cultures, which are good for digestion and are reported to promote growth in laboratory animals, are deader than plastic doornails.

But even the "all natural" yogurts which are flavored will typically have about 100 extra calories from the fruit syrup. As far as calories go, you might as well be eating a cup of yogurt into which you had mashed two-thirds of a chocolate candy bar! Now that I think of it, I'm surprised no one has yet put a chocolate-flavored yogurt product on the market — although I suppose that would spoil the image of yogurt as a health food. But if you want the blunt truth, there's no nutritional difference — in terms of calories or vitamins or anything else — between a fruit-flavored yogurt and a chocolate-flavored yogurt.

Yes, you say, but . . . *plain* yogurt? It's tasteless!

Well, taste is a relative thing. Not long ago, I felt the same way. But once I realized that fruit-flavored yogurt was loaded with sugar, I decided to give the plain variety an honest chance. At first, I simply put in some chopped fruit, sometimes running it through the blender, and that added maybe 20 calories or so, but a lot of taste and a lot of vitamins A and C. Did it taste sweet, like commercial yogurt? No, I admit it didn't. But after a while, it began to taste *better* than commercial yogurt. After a few weeks, it got to the point where commercial yogurt tasted sickeningly sweet, like a child's confection.

And believe it or not, in another few weeks I found that I was eating plain yogurt by itself and enjoying it. If that sounds a little difficult to believe, consider that to a person who's never drunk wine, a pale white wine tastes somewhere between dull and vaguely bitter. Sweet wines are almost always preferred at first, but eventually, even the most occasional wine drinker learns to prefer the dry wine that he once thought was insipid. So, you can *learn* to really enjoy plain yogurt, just as many people are learning to enjoy spring water instead of soda.

Actually, the way I enjoy yogurt most is to put about four ounces of the plain variety inside half a cantaloupe and add a heaping tablespoon of cottage cheese, which I blend with the yogurt. That whole delicious treat has a total of only about 185 to 200 calories, still significantly less than one carton of sweetened yogurt.

But yet — and this is an important point — the real purpose of eating natural yogurt with fresh fruit instead of the sweetened commercial product is *not* simply to shave off calories. The real purpose, as I see it, is to eat a *reasonable* number of calories in the most totally satisfying form. In other words, if you typically make a lunch out of sweetened yogurt and one or two pieces of fruit, the total calories involved are not at all excessive for lunch. But by using plain yogurt and eating it with cantaloupe, you are getting something that is going to be more chewable, more filling, and much more nutritious than the sweetened yogurt. For the person who makes her lunch out of sweetened yogurt and fruit, a good substitute for the apple and banana that might typically follow the yogurt would be a good, thick slice of homemade whole wheat bread, or a somewhat smaller piece of a banana nut loaf bread made with whole wheat pastry flour and smaller amounts of soy flour. The calories from that lunch are going to be about the same as they were before, but the protein, fiber, and mineral content will be considerably higher, and the whole affair will be a lot more interesting and satisfying.

Is meat a natural food? What could be more natural than a juicy piece of meat? High in protein, B vitamins, and iron, meat is one of the least processed foods we eat today. The one item that virtually all fast-food establishments feature is hamburgers, and if you go into an expensive restaurant you're likely to find the menu featuring the likes of steak *poivre* and rack of lamb. At home, the family of modest means eats meat loaf while the wealthy family dines on strip steak. Italians are fond of veal, Germans of sausage, the Greeks of lamb. Many of us are fond of all three, and a lot more beside.

Yet, there's something about meat — particularly beef — that many people regard as unnatural. If you go into a "natural foods" restaurant and ask for a steak, they'll look at you like you're mad. When the average person becomes interested in eating "health foods," one of the first things he's likely to do is to cut down on beef consumption. People worried about their hearts do the same thing. Marathon runners, who are a long way from having cholesterol problems, often say they avoid eating red meat because it makes them feel sluggish. Vegetarians will say that eating meat is morally unnatural. Some consumers will admit that meat is a natural food, but because cattle are often fattened with the use of hormones, their meat is chemically tainted and should be avoided as unnatural.

But all that still doesn't answer the question of whether or not meat in general and beef in particular are basically natural foods. Neither does it address the role of meat in the reducer's diet.

To cut through the confusion around the subject of meat, we

have to understand that there are basically two different kinds of meat: that which comes from wild animals and that which comes from domesticated animals. And the major difference between these two kinds of meat is the fat content.

The best examples of animals raised entirely in the natural state are marine creatures. Except for some pollution, the habitat, diet, and life-style of ocean creatures probably hasn't changed since the days of Noah. But history aside, virtually all fish have an extremely low fat content. Sea bass and halibut, for instance, have just a little over 1 percent fat content. Shrimp and squid have a tad *less* than 1 percent fat, while the abalone is only ½ of 1 percent fat. Crabs and mussels are about 3 percent fat, and terrapins just a little bit more. Tuna and swordfish hit the 4 percent fat level, while mackerel is quite extraordinary with 12 percent fat content.

Freshwater fish aren't much fatter, on the average. Catfish are only 3 percent fat, carp 4 percent, while the lake trout is 10 percent fat. From this little survey, you can see that even when you lightly brush on some butter before baking your fish, the fat content isn't going to average very much more than about 5 percent.

In greasy contrast, the edible portion of the carcass of a choice grade steer, the kind most frequently sold in supermarkets, contains 34 percent fat. The same meat from a prime grade animal is no less than 39 percent fat!

The reason for this enormous difference is not simply a reflection of a difference in species. Rather, it is the direct result of the way these animals are bred and raised. And the most prevalent technique for raising livestock is to make them grow as quickly as possible and reach a certain level of fatness.

To begin with, a serious breeder only breeds from stock which has already demonstrated its ability to get fat fast. The more marbling in the meat, the higher the "grade" of the animal. Second, at the end of the feeding periods, the animals are fed an extremely rich ration calculated to promote the most rapid possible growth. Third, the animals are discouraged — often prevented — from getting anything remotely resembling exercise. Exercise not only tends to make an animal tougher and leaner, reducing its market value, but burns up calories that would otherwise go to create poundage. Finally, synthetic hormones are sometimes used to speed weight gain even more. Because of laws which are still in a state of flux, and toxicity problems, some growers have turned away from synthetic hormones and are using what they call "natural" means of fattening. One "natural" method consists of inserting a spiked instrument resembling a small Christmas tree into the vagina of a heifer, which causes hormone and behavior changes and speeds growth. Other growers introduce a certain kind of bacteria into the animal's stomach, which enhances digestion and speeds growth. Sometimes heifers are spayed so they fatten like steers. How "natural" all that is I'll let you decide for yourself.

It's difficult to get accurate and truly comparable figures for the fat content of undomesticated animals resembling steers, but some preliminary information I've seen from analyses done on wild antelope and zebras indicates that these animals have only about one-quarter to one-third the fat content of domesticated beef. Even reindeer, which are probably carrying some extra fat to protect them against cold weather, have a fat content of only 15 percent.

From this perspective, it's reasonable to say that the modern domesticated steer is an unnatural creature, in the sense that it probably couldn't survive in its present form if turned out to the wild. If it *did* survive, it would be a lot leaner and tougher. Actually, the wild boars which are avidly hunted in some parts of the United States are the progeny of swine which escaped captivity years ago and became what are known as feral pigs. But their flesh is said to be so tough and rank as to be virtually inedible.

Chickens are usually considered to be less fatty than beef, and rightly so. A raw roasting chicken is only 18 percent fat, while a capon is 21 percent fat. There are no wild chickens flying around in the woods, but for the sake of comparison, the quail has a fat content of only 7 percent.

The rabbit is an animal which apparently has not been changed that much by breeding, so there isn't too dramatic a difference between the wild variety and the domesticated: 5 percent fat versus 8 percent.

Whether or not the fat-laden steer would be more healthful if it was somehow naturally fat instead of being forced into obesity, I can't say. But the question is only theoretical, because there is no animal alive — at least that I've been able to discover — that is able to find food, escape its enemies, and mate while hauling around up to 40 or 50 percent of its body weight in useless fat.

To a weight-reducer, the important thing about fat is that it is the most concentrated form of calories you could possibly eat. While eating a pound of sugar will only add a little more than half a pound to your weight, eating a pound of fat will add about one pound, five ounces of blubber.

Despite all that, I'm not going to suggest that you never eat meat again. Only that you eat it a little more thoughtfully.

While a good part of the extra fat content in beef is marbled throughout the flesh and is all but impossible to remove with a knife and a fork, many cuts of meat can be trimmed without difficulty. *For every ounce of fat you cut away, you're saving yourself about 250 calories of blubber-power.* By getting yourself into this one habit, you can eliminate anywhere from 500 to 1,500 calories a week, depending upon how much meat you eat.

When shopping for meat, spend a little more and buy only the leanest cuts. Think of it this way: that extra money you spend is buying you slenderness. Lean hamburger has only half the fat content of the regular grind, with the result that eating one lean burger instead of the regular kind will save you 60 calories. If the lean meat tastes a little dry (it shouldn't if you don't overcook it), you can moisten it with some slices of fresh tomato or a little ketchup. Whatever you do, though, don't use mayonnaise, which is practically pure fat itself.

The best way for a dieter to enjoy beef is to buy a very lean cut, like round steak, cut it up into small cubes if you can't buy it that way, and serve it in a beef and vegetable stew. Let it simmer until the meat becomes tender, and add a variety of herbs to enhance the flavor and general feeling of satisfaction. If you then cool it in the refrigerator, you can skim away surface fat and save still more calories.

When eating chicken, avoid the fat and go for the white meat from which the skin has been removed. That will reduce the fat content from about 20 percent down to only 5 percent.

Natural foods can be abused. When some people go on a natural-foods diet, they give up white bread, white sugar, soda, cake, candy, and fatty cuts of meat. Instead, they eat lots of warm whole wheat bread covered with butter, honey dripped by the tablespoon into cups of herb tea, glass after glass of fruit juice, cashews, walnuts, almonds, dried apricots, prunes, dates, figs, raisins, unhomogenized peanut butter, sunflower and pumpkin seeds, fruit and nut loaves loaded with oil and honey, and even "high protein" candy bars made with brown sugar instead of white. After a month of this, they get on the scale and discover they've gained two pounds and can't understand why.

And I say that from personal experience. Because at one time, that's exactly what I was eating — everything except the candy bars. I was even eating ice cream made from goat's milk and sweetened with honey and carob, under the self-inflicted delusion that "natural" calories didn't count.

We already talked about how commercial granola and flavored yogurt are little better than snack foods. But you can get into big trouble with many others traditionally regarded as health foods. Because along with their high density of nutrients, many also deliver a very high density of calories.

Dried fruits, long popular as health food items, are perfect examples. Among other good things, they're unusually high in vitamin A and iron, two nutrients which tend to be scarce in many diets and are especially difficult to get in "finger food." Great. So you stock your refrigerator with prunes, figs, dates, and dried apricots. And a couple of times every night, you raid your cache to get healthier and healthier.

But what some people seem to forget is that four prunes have 80 calories, four dates have 88 calories, four figs have 160 calories, and half a cup of dried apricots, 170 calories. You may even develop a taste for dried, sweetened pineapple, good for 180 calories a slice.

Don't get me wrong. With the exception of dried, candied pineapple slices — which ought not to be sold in health food stores at all — dried fruits really *are* good food. You could even call them health foods and I would never argue with that designation. Only I'd call them dangerous health foods for people like you and me who have an eating problem.

"Portion control!" a health-food-minded home economist exclaimed when I brought this subject up. "People have to learn portion control. They don't realize how much they're eating."

True enough. But when you've got a whole bagful of dried fruit sitting in your lap, "portion control" is easier said than done. So for people who enjoy dried fruit, I see two alternatives. The first is to be especially careful when eating it. Be aware that a single prune or a single date has more calories than a teaspoon of sugar. More important, be aware that eating a *handful* of prunes is like eating a small handful of sugar. Number two, never eat dried fruit from the bag. Take what you want to eat, go and sit down at the kitchen or dining room table, and eat your dried fruit slowly, savoring its good taste and appreciating its pleasant aroma. When you have finished, drink a nice, cool glass of water, which will sweep the sweetness from your mouth and signal the conclusion of eating.

You may find, however, that controlling your intake of dried fruit is extremely difficult. In that case, you can do what I did, and simply quit buying it. Instead, I buy fresh fruit, which contains all the nutrients of dried fruit plus the water that is naturally present in the fruit as well. Somehow my stomach is a lot more satisfied with half a cantaloupe than with four dates, even though they have the same number of calories. And while many times in the past I would grab a bag of figs and demolish at least eight of them in one or two minutes, I never find myself eating two entire cantaloupes, which I would have to do in order to get the same number of calories. And while before, it was easy for me to polish off half a cup of dried apricots (scarcely two ounces worth), I have yet to eat nine raw apricots at one sitting, which I would have to do to get the same calories.

Maybe what I'm saying is that we ought to redefine our idea of "health foods" to include fresh fruits of every kind as well as dried fruits. And that's certainly logical enough, since fresh fruit is more natural than dried fruit anyway.

With nuts, it's the same story. High in protein, B vitamins, iron, magnesium, and trace elements, nuts are also, unfortunately, very high in oil. A dozen roasted almonds, which you can easily polish off in the time between the end of the late news and the beginning of the "Tonight Show" is a 100-calorie snack. A mere quarter-cup of dried pecan halves is also worth better than 100 calories. So are ten peanuts roasted in the shell (technically, peanuts aren't nuts — they're legumes, but who cares?).

Walnuts have a very warm look and interesting texture, so many people use them for interior decoration, keeping a wooden bowl full of them on an otherwise empty table. But if you sit down in front of that little pile of edible decoration and take a nutcracker to ten of them, you've just ingested 264 calories. Which will not look nearly as pleasant on your thighs as they did on your table.

The grimmest statistic of all is one tablespoon of peanut butter: 94 calories. About the same as a tablespoon of mayonnaise and not that far behind a tablespoon of pure oil (120 calories). Now, commercial peanut butter is made with added fat and sugar, and the figure of 94 calories refers to the commercial variety. "Natural" peanut butter made with nothing but ground-up peanuts probably has somewhat fewer calories, although I haven't been able to find a reliable figure. But the caloric saving would come from not having the added fat, rather than from eliminating the sugar. In fact, adding sugar to peanut butter actually *cuts* the calorie count per tablespoon, because a tablespoon of peanut butter has twice as many calories as a tablespoon of plain white sugar. Remember, nothing — not even sugar — has the calorie-clout of oil.

Again, don't get the idea that I'm against nuts. If you eat them as food, instead of as crunchy little things to keep your mouth occupied, you're getting excellent nutrition. But exercise the same cautions I described for dealing with dried fruits. Never sit down with a can or a bag of nuts in front of you. Don't leave nuts lying around the house, shelled or unshelled. Realize that nuts are food, like meat, and should be given the same respect. As a matter of fact, many excellent vegetarian recipes call for nuts because of their high protein, vitamin, and mineral content. Incorporating them as an important part of a meal featuring grains or vegetables is probably the best way to enjoy the flavor and nutritional goodness of nuts.

There's no point, by the way, in buying "dry roasted" nuts in hopes of saving calories. There's already so much oil *inside* nuts that the small amount usually used in roasting them makes only a negligible difference. What I would suggest, though, is that you buy unsalted nuts. Besides being more healthful, unsalted nuts (like almost any unsalted food) do not inflame the appetite the way the salty kind do.

Ditto for sunflower and pumpkin seeds. Great health foods. Brimming with protein and vitamins — bursting with calories. Ounce for ounce, almost as many as peanut butter. Half an ounce of sunflower seeds would fit very nicely in the palm of your hand: you're looking at 80 calories. That's sunflower seeds that have already been hulled — the way nearly all of them are sold these days. But you can still get the unhulled variety in health food stores and I recommend those as a way of getting the good things that sunflower seeds have to offer without having to worry about eating too many too fast.

Two of the most venerable health foods are honey and brown sugar. Both, of course, are considered good "health foods" by dint of being substitutes for white sugar. Some nutritionists put down both of these products, pointing out that while a tablespoon of white sugar has only about 45 calories, a tablespoon of honey has about 65. And while brown sugar is considered more natural than the white product, the truth, they say, is that brown sugar is only minimally different from white.

Health food enthusiasts dismiss these allegations as counter-revolutionary propaganda, and claim the real reason nutritionists don't recommend them is they're "health foods" and nutritionists hate health foods.

The truth is that both parties are right. A tablespoon of honey does have about 20 more calories than a tablespoon of nasty old white sugar. A tablespoon of brown sugar has only about one calorie less than its albino brother, and is certainly no "health food." At the same time, though, to condemn these products for those reasons is somewhat misleading. And yes, if the truth be known, most nutritionists and dieticians *are* against health foods on religious grounds.

Personally, I feel that if you're going to have any sweeteners in your house at all, they ought to be honey and brown sugar, and here is why:

While honey is highly caloric, it does have two things in its favor. First, because it has much more flavor than sugar, many people learn to use much less honey in sweetening their food than they would sugar. Second, honey does have some interesting traces of nutrients which are not present in sugar. The difference isn't enormous, but so what? If people switch their money around from bank to bank to get one more half-percentage point of interest, why shouldn't you do the same thing with your food?

As for brown sugar, it's pretty much the same story. You'll probably tend to use a little less because it does have a flavor of its own, and most people would rather taste coffee or tea than brown sugar. Brown sugar is also more natural, and contains some of the trace elements found in the original sugar cane. One of them is chromium, which happens to be extremely important in helping the body metabolize sugar.

Having said all that, please keep in mind that calories from honey or brown sugar don't look any more healthful on you than calories from pig fat.

The proof of the natural pudding. While there are innumerable reasons why eating natural foods *ought* to help reduce your weight and keep you slender, proving it isn't all that easy. The one obstacle to carrying out a study which would prove or disprove my contention is that the majority of people who eat a diet emphasizing natural foods also get quite a bit of exercise, typically from activities associated with natural living: gardening, hiking, skiing, that sort of thing. They're also likely to be simply more conscious of their diet and their health in general. So it would be mighty difficult to find a group of people who are exactly like a "control group" in every respect except for their natural diet.

Based on my personal experience, though, I would say that eating natural foods is a definite factor in keeping your weight down. No, it's not foolproof. At the Wildwood Sanitarium in Georgia, operated by Seventh-Day Adventist medical missionaries, only vegetarian food is served, in keeping with the principles of their religion. So I was somewhat surprised when I discovered that one of the popular programs there was a reducing program. When I asked how it was possible for a vegetarian to become fat, the director of the program told me "it's easy. All you have to do is eat lots of bread, butter, cakes, cookies, and candy. And lots of oil on your salads."

On the other hand, although Seventh-Day Adventists are vegetarians, they do not have any special strictures against sugar or white flour. So most of those fattening foods mentioned aren't really "natural" in the sense that we are using the word here.

There is, however, a fascinating experiment we can look at to try to get an objective view of the relationship between natural foods and obesity. It was carried out by Michele Bremer, Ph. D., a nutritionist, and although published in abbreviated form in a nutrition journal, the complete study (actually done as her dissertation) has been published under the title of *An Examination of Some Aspects of Two American Diets* by The Soil and Health Foundation, Emmaus, Pennsylvania, 1975. What Bremer did was to feed a sizable number of test animals (mice and rats) two different diets, one composed of customary or "supermarket" foods and the other composed of only natural foods.

Half of the food used in the experiment was obtained from a well-known chain of restaurants which also manufactures frozen foods. That was called the "supermarket" diet. The other food was obtained from Fitness House, the corporate kitchen of Rodale Press, which, as Dr. Bremer puts it, is "generally regarded as the center of the natural-foods movement." Both groups of food were mixed into slurries, frozen, and fed to the animals to eat as they wished.

Here are some of the typical items which were included in the "supermarket" diet: cornflakes and milk, chicken pie, chocolate pudding, meat loaf, milk shake, hamburger, apple pie, Cool Whip, french fries, spaghetti and meatballs, Jell-o, Oreo cookies, beef TV dinner, hot dogs and beans, bologna and cheese sandwich, fillet of flounder, corn, vegetable soup, and canned fruit cocktail.

Here are some of the typical items included in the natural foods diet: granola with milk, brown rice, chili con carne, polenta (a cornmeal dish), salad, cashew-millet casserole, fruit, cheesecake, corn bread, rice-wheat kasha, cherry crisp, peanut butter, liver with bacon, and bananas with custard sauce.

After careful analysis of the contents, Dr. Bremer designed the diets in such a way that although they contained different foods, *the calorie count, ounce for ounce, was almost exactly the same.*

For a period of months, which is a very long time in the life of a mouse, the animals ate their respective diets. When the appointed hour came, as it does for all laboratory animals, a representative sample was chosen to be autopsied and analyzed. A special effort was made to select from the supermarket group only those animals which appeared to be healthy. (It turned out that during the course of the experiment, the animals eating the supermarket diet, although kept in the same laboratory, developed skin infections which most of the "natural food" animals resisted.)

The analysis revealed two facts of major importance. First, the supermarket group was considerably heavier than the natural foods group. Perhaps even more important, they had a sharp increase in percentage of body fat, indicating that their increased weight was not in the form of muscle or bone.

Second, at one point in the experiment — which was actually a series of experiments — both groups of animals were given access either to natural foods or supermarket foods. Almost without exception, the animals chose the supermarket foods, probably because they were sweeter. That observation is important, because it shows that even animals may select foods which are unhealthful.

Dr. Bremer told me about another interesting observation which was not included in her written report because it was not "scientific." She said that the man who was in charge of cleaning the animal cages told her that while the natural foods group permitted themselves to be handled during cleaning operations, the supermarket group was a very ill-tempered lot and exhibited frenzied and vicious behavior when their cages were being cleaned.

In another experiment, the same tests were repeated, using rats instead of mice. But in the rat group, the obesity difference for some reason was not found. However, the supermarket animals still had a higher percentage of body fat.

So make of it what you will. Are men more like mice or like rats? Or like neither? No real conclusion, I think, can be drawn from this study, but one finding which is at least highly suggestive is that in both instances, the animals eating what Dr. Bremer calls a "typical

American diet" had a higher percentage of body fat than animals fed natural foods. And health scientists today are putting much greater emphasis on this fat-percentage measurement than on the more simplistic one of mere weight.

12

Cooking to Cut the Calories and Keep the Flavor

by Sharon Faelten
Janice Worsham, research associate

You may be leary of spending too much time at the stove for fear that you'll end up looking like Buddha's twin brother. Ironically, giving some extra time — and careful attention — to cooking will actually *save* you calories.

The basic principle here is learning to recognize the real calorie enemies in your recipes — fat and sugar — so that by manipulating the ingredients, you can reduce the calorie total of many of your favorite dishes. In some instances, calorie savings will seem small. But you may be making up to a dozen small adjustments each day and several larger ones in the course of a week, resulting in a significant saving of calories.

Look for recipes that call for fresh ingredients. When they do not, use fresh anyway. Choosing to use only fresh ingredients optimizes every flavor and texture offered in a meal. In other words, make the most of what you are eating rather then eating the most of what you cook.

When fresh parsley is listed, for instance, *use* fresh parsley. When dehydrated parsley flakes are listed, again use fresh parsley. The pungency of this herb when fresh gives life to baked potatoes, Cornish hens, or steamed onions to a degree that cannot be approached by those stale flakes for sale in the "spice" section at the grocery store. The caloric difference is practically nil, and the flavor is tremendously enhanced.

Don't ignore calls for fresh-ground pepper in recipes. An old-fashioned pepper mill that grinds whole peppercorns can be a great aid in augmenting the flavor of meat and vegetables. It not only tastes more like pepper than the powder that's been pulverized and allowed to linger on the supermarket shelf for months, but adds a theatrical touch to meal preparation.

Potatoes present a glaring example of the flavor depletion in a whole food after it is processed and preserved. Mashed potatoes made from dehydrated potato flakes are a bogus form of the real thing. Both are made with added milk and butter, but with reconstituted flakes, most of the flavor comes from these two fatty ingredients alone. With fresh-mashed, you can cut down on milk and butter — and calories — and still enjoy a lot of real potato flavor.

All vegetables, in fact, should be fresh whenever possible. Home-frozen are next best; canned are the pits. And use of vegetables in soups is no exception. From time to time, a food editor will feature a "compost" or "garbage" soup stock utilizing a week's collection of household vegetable refuse, including soft spots cut from tomatoes and cucumbers or bruised, brown, lettuce leaves. This may be economical in dollars-and-cents, but it is a poor way to give flavor to your soup. A limp carrot or some wilted celery is okay, but in general, don't use an ingredient in soup that you would hesitate to serve in a salad or side dish.

Fresh ideas are as important as fresh ingredients. So first of all, sit down and *read* your cookbooks. Use recipes not as strict formulas but as guidelines to be improved upon. For instance, dieters have no use for recipes which call for "a can of cream of mushroom soup" as a cream sauce for vegetables or binder in a casserole. As a super-salty excuse for mushroom sauce, it will do nothing but overpower the honest, natural flavors of your food, prompting you to eat more in an attempt to satisfy your taste buds.

If your home library of cookbooks is nonexistent or inadequate, visit your town's public library and borrow two or three to get you started. A list of some helpful cookbooks appears at the conclusion of this section.

Optimizing flavor often requires less actual work in the kitchen, because the less you do to a food, the more likely it is to help control your weight. So look for *simple* recipes.

Desserts can be OK. Thinking about dessert is a good way to begin your new approach to less-fattening cooking, because desserts are some of the foods dieters have repeatedly been told they *must* sacrifice in order to escape permanent obesity. Not so. In fact, serving yourself something special and fun after supper may prevent those late-night attacks of "I-skipped-dessert-so-this-left-over-turkey-drumstick-won't-actually-set-me-back."

Break the rule of "no dessert" by searching your cookbooks for directions on steaming or poaching fruit, such as pears baked in wine. Or redesign some of your own family favorites.

Say your family loves apple pie. Making apple pie requires that you peel, core, and slice apples; sift and measure flour; cut in shortening (F-A-T); and roll and crimp the dough. If you delight in a fancy latticework cover, the entire process can take the better part of an hour.

On the other hand, just plain apples seem to be an inelegant dessert to set before company. *Why not just bake the apples*?

Baking somehow enhances the natural sweetness of ripe fruit and still produces something warm and yummy to serve steaming from the oven. Even with a sprinkle of brown sugar or a touch of honey, the total calories per serving are not more than 100, compared to over 300 for apple pie. Furthermore, it takes just seconds to set a corer to a few apples, compared to that precious hour spent fussing with pastry dough. The saved time is a bonus to the saved calories.

Desserts are a must if other members of your family can sit down and eat two pieces of cheesecake and not gain an ounce. The seeming unfairness of that is likely to breed feelings of hopelessness in you that will contribute toward possible failure of your weight-loss program. *But who can resist cheesecake?*

I can't. So I redesigned my favorite cheesecake recipe to yield nearly 200 fewer calories per serving than the original. The result not only tastes great *and* saves calories, but it gives you enough protein (17 grams per serving) to redeem it from being an empty-calorie food.

The original cheesecake had twice as many egg yolks, over a cup of sugar, twice as much cream cheese (at 850 calories per 8-ounce package), and regular creamed cottage cheese. Switching to uncreamed cottage cheese and doubling the amount still didn't catch up to the total calories in cream cheese. Wheat germ is equivalent to graham cracker crumbs calorically, and you may prefer a higher proportion of crumbs. Finally, substituting fresh fruit in the topping for the cherry-syrup filling in the original lopped another 150 calories off the total.

Sensible Sensual Cheesecake

Crust
1 cup raw wheat germ
1 cup fine graham cracker crumbs (7½ crackers)
⅓ cup melted butter

Combine. Reserve ¼ cup for topping. Press mixture into glass pie dish or lightly buttered 9-inch springform pan. Chill briefly until set.

Filling
4 ounces cream cheese
2 whole large eggs and white of another
2 cups (1 pound) low-fat cottage cheese
⅓ cup light honey
2 tablespoons instant nonfat dry milk powder
1 tablespoon fresh lemon juice
2 teaspoons vanilla

Combine in blender until smooth.

Topping
1 cup plain yogurt
1 tablespoon light honey
1 teaspoon vanilla

Mix thoroughly with fork until blended.

Pour filling into shell and bake in preheated 325° oven for 25 minutes. Remove, spread with topping and reserved crumbs, and return to oven for 10 minutes more.

Remove cheesecake from oven and place on a rack to cool. The center will still be watery, but will firm up during cooling. Chill well and top with fresh strawberries or blueberries before serving.

Yield: 8 servings (2 in. × 5 in. × 1½ in.). Generous, but realistic!

Calories: 373 per serving versus 555 for the original recipe.

What about those recipes for eggnog pie or Sacher torte you've collected at ladies' auxiliary bazaars? Or the chocolate souffle clipped from *Bon Appétit?* Or the strawberry chiffon pie shared with you by one of the guys in your Wednesday evening cooking class? Can they be salvaged?

Probably not. In certain cases, substitution or alteration of recipes will produce such pitiful results that you may become justifiably discouraged. Accept the fact that as long as there is a good angel in Weight-Control Heaven devising luscious low-calorie desserts, there will be a little red devil planting calorie traps like brandy Alexander pie.

Preparing meat and poultry. A major concern in your new approach to cooking will involve meat or poultry as the focal point of a meal. About half the meat sold for retail sale is industry-graded, based on tenderness, juiciness, and flavor. That is determined, among other things, by the amount of fat marbling in the cut, exclusive of trimmable fat. Meat sold at your butcher's or supermarket is probably either prime, choice, or good, with decreasing amounts of marbling respectively. Lesser-grade cuts have even less fat and if braised, can still taste flavorful and tender.

Table 1 compares caloric values for two grades of beef, both with and without trimmable fat.

Table 1. Beef cuts.

	CALORIES
CHUCK ROAST: 3½ oz., braised	
choice, lean and fat	289
choice, lean only	193
good, lean and fat	253
good, lean only	179
PORTERHOUSE STEAK: 3½ oz., broiled	
choice, lean and fat	465
choice, lean only	224
good, lean and fat	446
good, lean only	197

	CALORIES
T-BONE STEAK: 3½ oz., broiled	
choice, lean and fat	473
choice, lean only	223
good, lean and fat	442
good, lean only	199
RUMP ROAST: 3½ oz., roasted	
choice, lean and fat	347
choice, lean only	208
good, lean and fat	317
good, lean only	190

Frying meat — or poultry — means cooking in fat. That only burdens the food with extra calories. Your body does require a small amount of fat for good health. Save your "fat quota" for unheated polyunsaturated vegetable oils in salad dressings or a light spread of butter on your morning toast.

If your favorite recipe for meatballs calls for frying them first in some kind of fat, try these baked meatballs instead.

Casserole Meatballs

1 pound lean ground meat
1 egg
½ onion
1 clove garlic
2 tablespoons wheat germ
cayenne (just a sprinkle)
¼ teaspoon paprika
1 12-oz. can of tomatoes or tomato sauce
½ teaspoon basil

Combine the meat and egg. Grate the onion into the meat mixture. Put the garlic through a garlic press or mince it very finely into the mixture. Add the wheat germ, a sprinkling of cayenne, and the paprika. Shape into balls and place in a casserole. Pour the tomatoes and basil over the meatballs. Bake for an hour in a 350° oven or simmer on top of the stove for 50 to 60 minutes.

Yield: 4 to 6 servings.

Some weight-loss programs ban all pork and pork products from the diet. As Table 2 indicates, even trimming off excess fat doesn't lower the calories as much as it does with beef.

Table 2. Pork cuts.

	CALORIES
PORK LOIN: 3½ oz.	
lean and fat, roasted	387
lean only, roasted	254
lean and fat, broiled	418
lean only, broiled	270
HAM: 3½ oz.	
lean and fat, roasted	289
lean only, roasted	187
BACON	
2 medium slices, crisp	86

Poultry is a more favorable choice than beef or pork from a caloric standpoint. You may choose to remove the skin before stewing or roasting, which will cut some calories. (See Table 3.)

Table 3. Poultry.

	CALORIES		
	Fried	Roasted	Stewed
CHICKEN: 3½ oz.			
Light meat			
with skin	234	222	201
without skin	197	173	159
Dark meat			
with skin	263	253	233
without skin	220	205	192

	CALORIES		
	Fried	Roasted	Stewed
TURKEY: 3½ oz.			
Light meat			
with skin	*	187	*
without skin	*	152	*
Dark meat			
with skin	*	210	*
without skin	*	180	*

* values not available

Diced left-over turkey or chicken adds lean protein to Chinese-style stir-fry vegetables, adapted from a recipe in *The Green Thumb Cookbook* (Rodale Press, 1977).

Chop Suey

1 cup sliced onions
1 cup chopped celery
1 cup sliced green peppers
1 cup sliced mushrooms
1 to 2 cups mung bean sprouts
1½ tablespoons tamari soy sauce
1 to 1½ cups cooked, diced chicken or turkey
2 cups cooked brown rice
½ cup sliced or whole almonds

Saute onions and celery in small amount of oil for a few minutes, until onions are limp. Add peppers and mushrooms, cover, and heat thoroughly. Add the sprouts, tamari sauce, and chicken or turkey. Serve on brown rice and sprinkle with almonds.

Yield: 4 servings.

Fish and seafood in themselves are even lower in calories than meat or poultry, because they are relatively fat-free. Frying in breading and fat, drenching with butter, or smearing with tartar sauce, however, adds calories. (See Table 4.)

Table 4. Fish and seafood.

	PORTION	CALORIES
Bluefish, baked with butter	3 oz.	135
Clams, raw	4 or 5 clams	56
Cod, broiled with butter	3 oz.	145
Crab meat, deviled—prepared with bread cubes, butter, parsley, eggs, lemon juice, and catsup	3 oz.	160
Crab meat, steamed	1 cup	135
Fish sticks, breaded and cooked	3 sticks	150
Flounder, baked with butter	3 oz.	171
Haddock, baked or broiled without butter	3 oz.	66
Haddock, dipped in egg, milk, and bread crumbs, and fried	3 oz.	140
Halibut, broiled with butter	3 oz.	144
Lobster, cooked (no butter)	1 cup	138
Mackerel, broiled with butter	3 oz.	201
Oysters, fried	3 oz.	204
Oysters, stewed with condensed milk	1 cup	206
Perch, dipped in egg, milk, and bread crumbs, and fried	1 fillet	195
Salmon, baked or broiled with butter	3 oz.	156
Salmon, smoked	3 oz.	150
Scallops, breaded and fried	3 oz.	165
Scallops, steamed	3 oz.	95

	PORTION	CALORIES
Shad, baked with butter and bacon slices	3 oz.	171
Shrimp, breaded with egg, bread crumbs, and flour or batter, and french fried	3 oz.	192
Shrimp, cooked (canned)	3 oz.	99
Swordfish, broiled with butter	3 oz.	138
Tuna, canned in oil—drained	1 can (6½ oz.)	309
Tuna, canned in water	1 can (6½ oz.)	234
Tuna salad	1 cup	349

If you usually fry your fish, try poaching as an alternative. Or broil and serve with a fat-free lemon sauce.

Poached Fish*

1½ pounds fresh fish fillets
2 cups water
3 tablespoons white vinegar
¼ cup finely cut onions
3 whole peppercorns
2 sprigs fresh parsley or dill
1 bay leaf, crushed

Cut fish into 6 serving portions and place them in a large skillet. Combine all other ingredients and add to pan. Bring to a boil; cover pan and reduce heat to low. Simmer 6 to 8 minutes or until fish flakes easily with a fork. Lift fish out of liquid carefully with a pancake turner. Serve with lemon wedges.

Yield: 6 servings.

* From *The Art of Cooking for the Diabetic* by Katharine Middleton and Mary Abbott Hess (Chicago: Contemporary Books, 1978).

Lemon Sauce for Broiled Fish

3 tablespoons lemon juice
⅛ teaspoon dry mustard
¼ teaspoon basil

Place fish on lightly oiled broiler pan and baste with sauce. Lemon sauce adds about 5 calories per tablespoon to fish, compared to 74 calories per tablespoon of tartar sauce.

Serve vegetables often . . . and right. A glance at Table 5 will show that vegetables as they arrive from the produce market are caloric midgets. Used raw in salads or lightly steamed, they range only from about 10 to 95 calories per serving.

Table 5. Vegetables.

	PORTION	CALORIES
Asparagus	4 spears	12
Beans, green	½ cup	15
Beans, lima	½ cup	95
Beets	½ cup, diced	27
Broccoli	½ cup, diced	20
Brussels sprouts	½ cup	28
Cabbage, green	½ cup, shredded	15
Carrots	½ cup, grated	24
Cauliflower	½ cup	14
Corn	1 ear	70
Eggplant	½ cup, diced	19
Mushrooms	½ cup, sliced	10
Peas	½ cup	57
Spinach	½ cup	20
Tomatoes	1 medium	40
Zucchini	½ cup	13

But watch out — vegetables can be real wolves in sheeps' clothing when glazed, candied, smothered with hollandaise sauce, or drenched in Roquefort dressing. All these touches add fat or sugar — or both.

As with fruit, the less you do to vegetables, the lower the caloric value is likely to be. As a side dish, simmer just until tender and sprinkle with fresh-ground pepper or lemon juice. Examples are taken from *The Rodale Cookbook* (Rodale Press, 1973).

Skillet Asparagus

2 to 2½ pounds fresh asparagus
¼ cup lemon juice

Break or cut off tough ends of asparagus stalks. Wash asparagus tips thoroughly with cold water; if necessary, use a brush to remove grit.

Fill a large skillet with 1½ inches of cold water and bring to a boil. Add asparagus spears; cover and simmer for 10 to 12 minutes (depending on size and tenderness of asparagus) until it is easily pierced with a fork.

Remove skillet from heat and remove asparagus spears with slotted spoon to heated serving dish. Sprinkle with lemon juice.

Yield: 4 to 5 servings.

Steamed Penny Carrots

⅓ cup water
2 cups sliced carrots
½ teaspoon lemon juice
freshly chopped mint or parsley for garnish

In a small, heavy saucepan, bring ⅓ cup water to a boil over medium heat. Add sliced carrots and lemon juice. Cover tightly and simmer over low heat for 15 to 20 minutes or just until carrots are barely tender.

Remove from heat. Turn into serving dish, garnish with chopped mint or parsley, and serve.

Yield: 4 to 5 servings.

Potatoes — white and sweet — are higher in calories than most other vegetables, but you do not necessarily have to banish them from your kitchen kingdom. The more you interfere with the simple, unadulterated potato, the higher the calories will go. (See Table 6.)

Table 6. Potatoes.

	CALORIES
White	
1 large baked, plain	145
1 large, boiled in skin	173
1 cup mashed, using only milk	137
1 cup mashed, using milk and butter	198
10 french fries, 3½ in.-4 in.	214
1 cup pan-fried	456
Sweet	
1 medium baked, plain	161
1 medium, candied	286

Salads without fatty dressings. Needless to say, there are no "recipes" for salads. Experiment freely. Two or more greens are more interesting than one. For example, buttercrunch lettuce, raw spinach leaves, and shredded red cabbage give contrast of flavor, texture, and color. Make a point of using what is in season in your area for optimum freshness.

Prepare only the amount of greens you plan to use in the next meal — a generous handful per person. Wash thoroughly and drain it well in a wire basket or on a clean, absorbent towel. Refrigerate, covered, for crispness while you prepare the rest of the meal. Just before mixing the salad, tear the greens into bite-size pieces.

At that point, the list of possible additions is practically infinite. To give you a good idea of the variety of salad ingredients you can use, let's spread out some of our favorites: apples (diced), artichoke hearts, raw or cooked beans (green, wax), beets (slices or shredded), beet greens, broccoli, cabbage (red, savoy, Chinese), carrots, cauliflower, celery, chick peas, chicory, cucumbers, dandelions, endive, fennel, garbanzos (chick peas), garlic, grapefruit, grapes, kale, kidney beans, mint, mushrooms, mustard greens, onions, parsley, peas, peppers, radishes, scallions, spinach, sprouts, squash (summer), tomatoes, turnip greens, water chestnuts, watercress, and zucchini.

Cottage cheese and grated cheese are more economical salad additions than Cheddar, calorie-wise. One tablespoon of grated Parmesan tossed throughout the salad adds a lot of cheese flavor and only 25 calories. One tablespoon of uncreamed cottage cheese adds only 8. By comparison, a cubic inch of Cheddar cheese adds 68.

If you love hard-boiled eggs on your salad, use just the whites and save yourself 65 calories per egg. If you relish crisp fried croutons, add half a slice of toasted whole wheat bread, diced, and eliminate still more fat and calories.

A salad is a dieter's Garden of Eden until the dressings are poured on. Not only does excess dressing mean excess calories, it also makes the salad limp, soggy, and unappealing. To minimize the amount of dressing necessary to dress your salad, mix it in an oversize bowl, large enough to toss the salad freely and thoroughly distribute the dressing. To add more flavor to the salad, rub the inside of the bowl with a split clove of garlic.

When dressing a salad, remember that by sticking to oil-and-vinegar-plus-herb dressings, you avoid the sugar and extra fat of cream and egg yolks in creamy dressings. With oil-and-vinegar-base dressings, the classic proportions of three or four parts oil to one part vinegar can be reduced to two to one. You may even dare to try a one to one ratio for further fat reduction.

The cructs sold along with foil envelopes of powdered salad dressing mixes are graduated for specific amounts of water, vinegar, and oil. You don't have to adhere strictly to those demarcations. You're not developing film! By replacing just one tablespoon of oil with the same amount of vinegar or water per batch of dressing, you will save yourself 30 calories per salad (assuming you use approximately ¼ cup of dressing each time). If you eat four salads in a week, that's 120 fewer calories.

Carry this approach over to your own favorite recipes for oil-and-vinegar dressings.

If you really *love* creamy dressings, you can still have them — if you make them yourself. The sugar and fat (from cream or egg yolks) in your recipes will push the calorie count up to "tilt" on an otherwise low-calorie course of green and raw vegetables, so scour your cookbooks for recipes that lend themselves to some minor adjustments. Yogurt-based dressings such as the following add plenty of zest and very few calories to your salad.

Green Onion Dressing

1 cup plain yogurt
¼ to ⅓ cup thinly sliced green onions
2 tablespoons fresh lemon juice
fresh-ground black pepper to taste

Combine ingredients and serve chilled.
Yield: approximately 1¼ cups.
Calories: about 9 per tablespoon.

Eggless mayonnaise, at just 20 calories per tablespoon, can be used as the base for Russian dressing. It's especially useful to those who are watching cholesterol *and* calories.

Eggless Mayonnaise

1 cup low-fat cottage cheese
2 tablespoons oil
1 tablespoon water
1 tablespoon cider vinegar
1 teaspoon dry mustard
½ teaspoon paprika
dash pepper

Blend all ingredients together in blender until smooth, occasionally stopping to scrape sides with rubber spatula. Thin with extra water if necessary. Cover and refrigerate for up to one week before use.

For Russian-style dressing, add 1 tablespoon or more of catsup to above. Additional calorie count will be negligible.

Yield: 1 cup, at 28 calories per tablespoon.

In comparison, most commercial salad dressings average about 75 calories per tablespoon.

By the way, your blender can be your best friend. With it, you can achieve a creamy consistency otherwise possible only with copious amounts of cream, eggs, and/or oil. An electric rotary-beater mixer just won't do. With a blender, it takes just seconds to produce what several minutes of high-speed beating can only attempt to achieve.

We tried our new approach to cooking to find a suitable alternative to creamed cottage cheese, which weighs in at 235 calories per cup. By buying the dry, uncreamed cottage cheese and creaming it ourselves, we eliminated 100 calories. And the flavor compares favorably with the bought creamed cottage cheese.

Home-Creamed Cottage Cheese

Add 2 tablespoons nonfat or skim milk to 1 cup of dry, uncreamed cottage cheese and flash-blend (that is, blend only for a second).

Net calories: 135.

Sauces for a slender gander. Meat sauces and gravies are obviously just cloaks of fat. Why trim fat from a slab of roast beef or peel skin from chicken, only to replace it with gravy? Low-fat sauces aren't all that easy to make, but they aren't impossible, either.

The technique of reduced-fat sauces has been perfected by the French chef Michel Guérard, and many variations on that technique are described fully in his book, *Michel Guérard's Cuisine Minceur* (Bantam Books, 1977). The basis for such sauces is a meat stock prepared by first carefully trimming the meat of excess fat. The meat is browned slowly (without added fat), then covered with water. Vegetables and herbs are added, and it is simmered gently, partially covered, over low heat for about three hours, or until the meat is done. From time to time, any fat which rises to the surface is skimmed off.

The stock is strained through a fine-mesh strainer to obtain as pure a broth as possible. After it cools to room temperature, the stock is refrigerated for several hours or overnight. Any remaining hardened fat appearing on the surface is again removed.

The stock is then reduced (made more concentrated) by additional simmering or is sometimes thickened with a binder, such as arrowroot.

In many recipes, such reduced cooking liquids are combined with vegetable purées to achieve sauces for vegetables, meat, and seafood. The sauces may also be completed with a combination of ricotta cheese and yogurt called *fromage blanc* (white cheese), as in Monsieur Guérard's parsley sauce. It's great as gravy on mashed potatoes!

Parsley Sauce

large bunch of parsley
2 shallots, peeled and finely minced
1 cup of stock (to serve with meat, use veal stock; to serve with seafood, use fish stock)
2 teaspoons mushroom purée } directions follow
2 tablespoons *fromage blanc* }
lemon juice
pepper

Remove all the stems from the parsley. In a saucepan, cook together over low heat the parsley sprigs, shallots, and stock for 15 minutes. Strain the mixture and reserve the broth. In a blender, combine the parsley, shallots, mushroom purée, *fromage blanc* and a few drops of lemon juice. Blend well, thinning the purée with some of the stock.

Keep warm until served or store in refrigerator until needed.

Yield: 1¼ cups.

Fromage Blanc

low-fat ricotta cheese (be sure it is fresh; check sale date)
low-fat yogurt

Use either 1½ cups of ricotta and 4 tablespoons of yogurt or 2 cups of ricotta and 5 tablespoons of yogurt.

Combine in blender and mix until very smooth.

We suggest that you prepare a quantity of mushroom purée and refrigerate it for occasional use in sauces. Freeze a portion of this amount if you do not plan to use it often.

Mushroom Purée

1 pound fresh mushrooms, trimmed
1 tablespoon lemon juice
3 cups water
1 cup nonfat dry milk
pinch of pepper
touch of freshly grated nutmeg

Trim off any gritty ends of the mushroom stems. Rinse mushrooms well in cold water and drain in a colander. Roll them in lemon juice in a bowl to prevent them from darkening. Slice each mushroom in half.

In a saucepan, heat water and add the mushrooms, pepper, and nutmeg. Simmer over low heat, uncovered, for about 10 minutes, then stir in the nonfat dry milk. Simmer another 5 minutes, or until the mushrooms are tender.

Drain the mushrooms, reserving the cooking liquid. Purée in blender until smooth, thinning with from ¼ cup to ½ cup of the reserved liquid.

Keep warm over hot water, or refrigerate or freeze until needed.

Yield: 1⅔ cups.

The next time you serve turkey or chicken, take a closer look at your recipe for cranberry sauce. Mine called for two cups of sugar to a one-pound bag of cranberries. You can reduce the calories considerably by cutting way down on the sugar or substituting about half as much honey for each 4½ cups of whole berries — the yield from one bag. (I added a chopped apple both to compensate for some of the reduced sweetening and to add a less-tart flavor to the cranberries.)

Your own taste for sweetness will dictate the exact proportions of berries and sweetener that you use.

Cranberry Sauce

Original: strained of extra water (4 cups)	Calories
1 pound fresh berries (4½ cups whole, 4 cups chopped)	200
2 cups sugar	1,540
2 cups water	0
Total calories:	1,740
Calories per cup:	435
Calories per ½-cup serving:	218

Revised: not strained (3 cups)	Calories
1 pound fresh berries (4½ cups whole, 4 cups chopped)	200
½ cup honey	515
or	
⅔ cup sugar	513
1 cup apple, chopped	80
1 cup water	0
Total calories:	795
Calories per cup:	265
Calories per ½-cup serving:	132

Note: Commercial cranberry sauce falls slightly below standard recipe values at 404 calories per cup, 202 calories per ½-cup serving.

Combine all ingredients in saucepan. Cover and bring to boil over moderate heat. Uncover and simmer for 5 minutes. Remove from heat and allow to cool and thicken, then refrigerate.

The original recipe will probably have to be strained of some of the excess water.

Soup without grease. *Soups, like vegetables, are very innocuous as long as the amount of fat is controlled.* For soups based on meat or poultry stock, prepare the broth a day in advance and refrigerate. Then be sure to skim all the solidified fat from the surface of the chilled stock before adding the other ingredients for soup. (Use essentially the same procedure described earlier for preparing low-fat stocks.) Add as many vegetables as you wish. Remember, however, that beans and legumes are higher in calories and consequently will up the total for your soup.

Think of soup instead of hot cocoa when you come in from ice-skating or shoveling snow. A mug of steaming, velvety tomato bouillon has about 45 calories compared to 243 for a cup of homemade cocoa with milk. Hot tomato bouillon, from *The Rodale Cookbook,* will fill you up without filling you out.

Tomato Bouillon

4 cups tomato juice
1 bay leaf
1 small onion, studded with whole cloves
1 stalk celery, with leaves
3 peppercorns
4 cups chicken or beef broth
chopped parsley for garnish
yogurt (served separately)

In large pot, combine tomato juice, bay leaf, onion with cloves, celery, and peppercorns. Slowly bring to a boil. Reduce heat and simmer for half an hour.

Remove soup from heat and strain. Add broth and place over medium heat. Simmer for 15 additional minutes.

Serve with chopped parsley and plain yogurt.

Yield: approximately 8 cups.

Calories: 45 calories per cup.

Cream soups are in the same league with creamy salad dressings unless special efforts are made to avoid the cream, which is 38 percent fat. However, a creamy effect can be achieved by puréeing a stock-and-vegetable soup in your blender. Try this the next time you make cream of potato, cream of mushroom, or cream of celery soup: omit the cream, use extra amounts of the vegetable (cooked until soft enough to purée easily), and blend with hot stock and a few tablespoons of instant nonfat dry milk until smooth. Small sprigs of fresh parsley are an excellent garnish for cream-style soups.

Break your fast, not your reducing program. Skipping breakfast is a coward's way of avoiding fried eggs, bacon, and buttered toast. If you enjoy your eggs sunny-side up, cooking them in steam instead of fat will save you calories. Or try the double-boiler method for scrambled eggs.

Steam-Fried Eggs

Heat moderately a frying pan for which you have a close-fitting lid. Brush very lightly with butter. Break eggs into the pan. Add 2 tablespoons water or milk.

Cover the pan and cook over very low heat until the whites are firm — 8 to 10 minutes. Sprinkle with a little fresh-ground pepper or paprika.

Scrambled Eggs

Heat water in the bottom part of a double boiler.

Beat as many eggs as you wish, using one tablespoon of water per egg.

Brush the upper part of the double boiler very lightly with butter.

Add the eggs and scramble them with a fork or wire whisk. (This takes slightly longer than the frying-pan method.)

Nitrites used as preservatives in bacon, plus its high fat content (52 percent) make it a doubtful item for a healthful breakfast. However, if you feel that Sunday mornings are a complete vacuum without bacon and eggs and the morning paper, use lean bacon, broil (not pan-fry) until crisp, and drain thoroughly on paper towels before setting them beside your sunny-side ups. Some research indicates that vitamin C sharply decreases the level of harmful nitrosamine formation by nitrites in the digestive tract, so a big glass of orange juice may counteract some of bacon's evil effects.

Breaking the bacon-and-egg habit may benefit your calorie-cutting plans at breakfast. A large bowl of oatmeal, even with whole milk, has 200 calories. Sprinkled with cinnamon and sweetened with a tablespoon of honey, the total is 265. And it will probably be more filling and satisfying to your stomach than a couple of scrambled eggs, two slices of bacon, and lightly buttered white toast, which provides 420 calories.

Kitchen math. Learn to cook with a pen as well as a spatula. In other words, cutting calories is not so much a matter of kitchen magic as kitchen math. Because those unnecessary calories are most likely to come from fat or sugar, the substitutions suggested in Table 7 may be a helpful guide to revising both new recipes and family specialties.

Table 7. Calorie-saving substitutions.

WHAT TO AVOID:	CALORIES	WHAT TO SUBSTITUTE:	CALORIES
Sour cream		Plain yogurt	
1 cup	495	Whole milk—1 cup	152
1 tablespoon	25	Skim milk, 1 cup	113
		Whole milk, 1 tablespoon	9
		Skim milk, 1 tablespoon	7
Sugar, white or brown		Honey (about twice the	
1 cup	770	sweetening power of sugar)	
1 tablespoon	46	½ cup	515
1 teaspoon	15	½ tablespoon	32
		½ teaspoon	11
		(Vanilla extract: In some recipes, the addition of ½ to 1 teaspoon of vanilla extract can increase "sweetness" because of the concentrated flavor. Eight calories per teaspoon.)	
Creamed cottage cheese		Uncreamed cottage cheese	
1 cup	235	1 cup	125
		Home-creamed cottage cheese	
		1 cup	135
Eggs, 3 whole (large)	246	Eggs, 2 whole (large) plus white only of a third	180

Table 8. Condiments.

	CALORIES (per tablespoon)
Barbecue sauce	23
Catsup	16
Chili sauce	16
Horseradish, prepared	6
Lemon juice, fresh	4
Mayonnaise	101
Mustard, prepared	15
Pickle relish, sweet	21
Seafood cocktail sauce	22
Soy sauce	12
Steak sauce	21
Tartar sauce	74
Vinegar	2
Worcestershire sauce	12

Values cited in this chapter are based on data in the following:

Kraus, Barbara, *Calories and Carbohydrates,* New York: Grosset & Dunlap, 1971.

Unpublished data, Consumer and Food Economics Institute, USDA.

USDA Handbook No. 8, *Composition of Foods,* December, 1963.

USDA Handbook No. 456, *Nutritive Value of American Foods in Common Units,* November, 1975.

USDA Home and Garden Bulletin No. 72, *Nutritive Value of Foods,* April, 1977.

AN ANNOTATED BIBLIOGRAPHY OF COOKBOOKS

This brief list is only a sampling of the many cookbooks which can be used in your approach to cutting calories in meal preparation. Each either provides many all-purpose recipes, emphasizes natural foods, or focuses on a specific — such as yogurt, use of herbs, or protein sources.

Survey several cookbooks in your library or bookstore to judge which best suit your food needs and tastes.

Albright, Nancy. *The Rodale Cookbook.* Emmaus, Pennsylvania: Rodale Press, 1973.

The introduction to this volume gives helpful advice for buying, storing, and cooking with ingredients such as herbs, seeds, yogurt, and whole grains. The section on beverages offers alternatives to soft drinks. The variety of soups includes purées, which rival cream soups.

Clamp, Betty Ann. *Cooking with Low-Cost Proteins.* New York: Arco Publishing Co., 1976.

Includes a fair-sized section on tofu (soybean curd), variations on fish salads, a nonfat marinade for fish steaks, and tables of nutritive values of beef, fish, grains, nuts, and seeds. Very useful to the nutrition-conscious dieter.

Editors of *Woman's Day. Woman's Day Cooking for Two.* New York: Random House, Fawcett Publications, 1976.

Preparing exactly what you need for two, thereby *planning* to avoid waste rather than *eating* to avoid waste.

Guérard, Michel. *Michel Guérard's Cuisine Minceur.* New York: Bantam Books, 1977.

An alternative to French high-calorie haute cuisine for the weight-conscious cook.

Hewitt, Jean. *The New York Times Natural Foods Cookbook.* New York: Quadrangle Books, 1971.

Similar in scope and philosophy to *The Rodale Cookbook.*

Hobson, Phyllis. *Making Homemade Soups and Stews.* Charlotte, Vermont: Garden Way Publishing, 1977.

An excellent guide to nutritious and flavorful soup-making, including defatted meat stocks and fat-free fish and vegetable stocks. Suggests use of stock as part of milk in cream sauces and gravies. Encourages experimentation and free substitution among ingredients.

Moyer, Anne. *The Green Thumb Cookbook.* Emmaus, Pennsylvania: Rodale Press, 1977.

You'll never serve soggy canned carrots again! Variety here is considerable — 350 recipes for over 61 different vegetables. You're sure to find several you like.

Rombauer, Irma S. and Brecker, Marion Rombauer. *Joy of Cooking.* Indianapolis, Indiana: Bobbs-Merrill Co., 1975.

The scope of *Joy of Cooking* qualifies it as a vital tool for all-purpose meal planning. Much variety without getting too exotic. Recipes easily lend themselves to alteration.

Robertson, Laurel; Flinders, Carol; and Godfrey, Bionwen. *Laurel's Kitchen, A Handbook for Vegetarian Cookery and Nutrition.* Berkeley, California: Nilgiri Press, 1976.

Advocating a variety of whole foods in moderation, it also includes a small section on weight control. Its wealth of nutrient information makes it a food manual as well as a recipe book.

Ross, Shirley. *The Seafood Book.* New York: McGraw-Hill Book Co., 1978.

How to buy and prepare every variety of fish and shellfish. Ignore instructions for frying; plenty are given for steaming, poaching, and broiling.

Truax, Carol. *The Woman's Day Book of Thin Italian Cooking.* Boston: Houghton Mifflin Co., 1978.

The author asserts that to eat Italian food and lose weight is a real miracle. How is that miracle possible? The herbs that make authentic Italian cuisine distinct have zero calories, and they are artfully used to bring out the most in each recipe. The number of calories is listed for each dish and for complete menus. Still another book which emphasizes using fresh ingredients; broiling, baking, or poaching instead of frying; and defatting stocks.

Whyte, Karen Cross. *The Complete Yogurt Cookbook.* San Francisco: Troubador Press, 1970. New York: Ballantine, 1976 (paperback).

Use of yogurt in such traditional high-calorie dishes such as dips, snacks, and spreads; even a low-calorie sherbet.

13

Shopping Wisely

Your behavior while marketing is critically important for two reasons.

First, it's difficult to eat food that you don't buy — unless you receive Care packages. Difficult, but not impossible, because in fact, most of us do from time to time get "Care packages" from relatives and neighbors. Usually cake or cookies. Then too, we may be eating 20 or 30 percent or even more of our daily diet outside the home. But still, for most people, home is where the food is.

The second reason that marketing is so important is that most people find it much easier to select their food wisely when it's sitting on a shelf or in the store freezer than when it's in their own refrigerator or in a bowl on the dining room table.

But that doesn't mean it's easy to get out of the supermarket carrying only the foods which in your most conscious moments you would choose to ingest and have become a part of your body. In fact, it becomes more and more difficult each year: the supermarkets go to great pains to take care of that. And too often, we play right into their hands.

In your typical supermarket, for instance, you will probably find more different kinds of soda than you will of all fresh fruits and vegetables put together. You might easily find 30 or 40 different kinds of cookies and 20 different kinds of crackers; if you can find one kind of whole wheat flour, you're lucky. If you have to go to a section of your supermarket that carries infant needs, you'll probably be forced to pass a gigantic candy and snack food section. In the supermarket closest to my house, you can't go to the area where such staples as eggs and butter are sold without passing a huge bakery section and rack after rack of pretzels, potato chips, and corn chips.

In that same market, the shopper looking to buy some frozen vegetables will be forced to take in a long eyeful of every imaginable kind of frozen cake and pie, all of them beckoning "buy me!" with gorgeous color photographs.

I'm told that in Boston, and maybe in other cities, there are supermarkets given over entirely to liquor, beer, and wine. At the rate things are going, I wouldn't be very surprised if whole supermarkets are soon given over to nothing but snack foods. In a sense, we already have something like that, because the total number of *all* food products sold in the corner grocery where I grew up did not even approach the number of snack and junk food items found today in a typical supermarket.

Probably, though, most people would resist the idea of going into a snack food supermarket. Indeed, according to one report I've seen, most people have no intention whatsoever of buying a lot of snack foods when they visit *any* supermarket: 78 percent of shoppers said their snack food purchases were made strictly on impulse. While the manufacturers of these products argue that they're only providing what people want, it's clear to me that there's a big difference between wanting something in a very conscious way, and deciding to buy it on an impulse.

Supermarkets, of course, do everything possible to try to encourage such impulse buying. Junk food is often placed in the immediate vicinity of staples. Large end-of-aisle displays most typically feature soda, cookies, crackers, marshmallows, etc. Walk down the aisle where fruit is sold and you may find that every 15 feet there is a big jumbled display of candy. That's a double trap: they're selling you candy when you're shopping for fruit or vegetables, and cashing in on the fact that people are more likely to buy candy when it's offered in a big jumble than they are when it's neatly stacked on the shelf. Now that I think of it, it's a triple trap, because the goodies on display are exactly at eye-level with a five- or six-year-old child.

But you aren't even safe when you're in the check-out line, because there you're apt to find more eye-level displays where cranky kids can reach out and ease their boredom with candy bars. Adults, too, are apt to be tired and hungry by the time they reach the check-out counter and are not above munching on a candy bar to soothe themselves.

Even in "health food" stores you're likely to find the area around the cash register covered with all kinds of candy bars and confections. The fact that they're made with honey or brown sugar instead of white sugar is no saving grace to the person with a weight problem. At the health food store where I often do some shopping, the candy bars are on one side of the cash register, and on the other side, gallons of ice cream and jars of fresh-ground peanut butter.

Girding your loins. At our workshop sessions, everyone agreed it's poor strategy to go shopping when you haven't eaten for several hours or more. Shopping when you're hungry only adds the force of true biological hunger to all the hidden and not-so-hidden persuaders that the supermarket has engineered to sell you "fun" foods which you had no intention of purchasing. Fighting off biology *and* psychology at the same time is no easy trick!

Yet, three out of four of our workshop participants admitted that they *did* shop when they were hungry — usually right after work. Here is a classic example of how the force of habit — sheer habit — pushes you toward overweight even when you realize full well what's going on.

Equally as unwise, maybe even more so, is shopping on Saturday afternoon after you've spent all morning running around from one store to another. You're hungry, your blood sugar is low, and you're so fatigued that you're almost dizzy. Shopping in that condition not only lowers your resistance to junk food, but might even give you the idea that you *deserve* some nice, rich goo as a reward for having run yourself ragged. Somehow, it never occurs to us that what we're *really* saying is: "I've been working so hard that I deserve to get just a little bit fatter."

Resolve right now that if you do fall into any of the patterns we've described, from here on in you're going to shop only after you've eaten a solid meal. My guess is that the best time of all is early in the day, so consider doing your marketing after eating a hearty breakfast on Saturday morning.

By now, it has probably occurred to you that it would be a good idea to take a shopping list into the market and buy only what you've decided — in your most rational mind — that you really want. I agree that lists are a good idea, and I urge you to try making a list for at least a few weeks. You may find that it will not only help you avoid unwanted snack items, but encourage you to buy more of what you would truly like to be eating — items like fresh fruits and vegetables, salad greens, cottage cheese, and fish.

Another benefit of shopping with a list is that you can buy all the ingredients you need to make new recipes. And making new recipes is a fine idea for anyone trying to improve their eating behavior. For one thing, it's a positive, pleasantly challenging way to break out of habitual eating patterns (like spaghetti and meatballs and garlic bread dripping with butter every Wednesday night). Creating new dishes also makes you more sensitive to the taste, texture, and aroma of food, which — although it may be surprising — is actually a good way to help gain control of your eating. That's because a great bulk of our overeating is not done with strange or new foods, but with the most familiar items — french fries, chocolate chip ice cream, pretzels, and so forth. But not having one or two key ingredients, I've found, is a common barrier to creating exciting new dishes. That's where your food list (and a couple of good cookbooks) can save your day.

The last thing I want to say about lists is that you should have one or two snack items on it to keep the list realistic and to remind yourself that you aren't *depriving* yourself of all snacks. And think for a while before deciding what snacks you want on that list. They should be foods that have a very enjoyable taste and that — if possible — leave you with a satisfied feeling. Pretzels would be a good example of a snack that will appear on very few lists indeed. Have you ever said — or heard anyone else say — "Wow, what delicious pretzels!"? They aren't very satisfying, either. In fact, because they're so salty, they also encourage you to drink soda or beer. The same goes for potato chips. On the other hand, if you really love brownies, decide ahead of time that you are going to buy two or three and really enjoy one with a glass of milk or a cup of coffee twice a week.

It's quite possible that after a month or two of your new eating behavior, you may not really want any snacks other than something like hard, juicy apples when they're in season or a plump honeydew melon. But if you've been accustomed to eating quite a few snacks, you'll probably find that your new program will be more successful if you don't give up all your snacks "cold turkey."

Having said that you should select the snacks you enjoy the very most, and despite the fact that the Prevention System of Weight Control does not tell you what to eat and what not to eat, I'm nevertheless going to list a group of snack items which I think you ought to at least *consider* never buying at all. They are:

chocolate chip cookies
marshmallow cookies
fig cookies
macaroons
pretzels
potato chips
corn chips
peanut butter and cheese cracker "sandwiches"
candy
soda

What makes these particular snack items so unwelcome? Two things: First, they are little hand grenades of calories, with one lumpy macaroon packed with 90 of them, and one chocolate chip cookie with 51. Second, there is something about these items that makes it difficult to quit eating them once you have started. Third, with the exception of the fig bars, they are junk food, unpure and simple.

Your personal danger foods. There are probably other items that you shouldn't buy at all, but only *you* know which they are. They are the foods which you simply can't resist and either gorge on or nibble constantly. Take peanuts, for example. Theoretically, they are a fine food for almost anyone: high in protein, unprocessed, free of sugar, and good tasting, they also come naturally in small sizes and keep without spoiling a long time, so that it's easy to just eat a few. Alas, all that is only true *theoretically.* For me, at least, a bag or a can of peanuts is nothing but a fat-producing machine. Because I *can't* eat just a few of them. For years, whenever they were in the house, I would grab them at about ten or eleven o'clock at night and eat them until my stomach almost ached. For the last year, peanuts have been on my *never* list.

Because I have very little self-control when it comes to food which is sitting in front of me, there are *lots* of items that I reject right at the supermarket, where, luckily, the temptation to buy them is only about 1 percent as strong as the temptation to eat them when they're on the kitchen counter or in the refrigerator. These items include just about all kinds of dried fruits — apples, pears, apricots, figs, dates, even raisins — except prunes, which for some reason I am able to eat with some semblance of rationality. I even avoid buying grapes, because experience tells me that I'm going to eat them until my stomach hurts.

Just as you will have to decide what foods to exclude completely from your shopping list, you can also choose the snack foods that you bring home for yourself or for your family partly on the basis of your ability to control yourself when eating them. If you know, for instance, that you can sit down and eat three or four walnuts and be done with them, then walnuts might be a fine, nutritious snack for you. If your family loves strudel, and you can enjoy and be satisfied with a two-inch slice a couple of times a week, then there's no reason why you shouldn't buy strudel. At the same time, reflection may reveal that something which many other people find quite innocuous — like English muffins, for example — are for you an irresistible snack.

Self-inquiry like the above can also be applied to food items which are not usually thought of as snacks. For some people, cold cuts and delicatessen items like sliced ham or potato salad are strictly "meal" foods. But reflection may reveal that for you, they are not only meal foods, but compulsive snacking items, too. Do you get an irresistible urge to make a salami and cheese sandwich at eleven o'clock at night when you know those foods are in the refrigerator? Is a 400-calorie wallop like that a reasonable part of your daily diet? Think about those questions and then decide if perhaps you would be better off not buying them at all.

I picked delicatessen items to illustrate this principle for a good reason: in general, foods sold in that section of your supermarket are high in price, high in preservatives, high in salt, and high in fat. They also perish quickly — which encourages you to eat them quickly.

For many people, the greatest challenge in shopping is posed by the fact that they are shopping not only for themselves, but for the rest of their family. What do you do when other family members (who may or may not have eating-behavior problems) expect you to bring home cupcakes, ice cream, potato chips, and other snacks you have a weakness for?

Many people will find that situation a convenient excuse to bring home junk food, telling themselves that it's for someone else, when they know perfectly well *they* are going to overeat on the snacks. And I don't say that self-righteously, either, because I used to do it all the time. I'd buy Fig Newtons and tell myself that they were relatively healthful snacks for the kids because of the figs, never admitting that I ate twice as many of them as they did. It was the same with ice cream, only more blatant: I used to "buy it for them," but somehow, I always managed to select flavors I liked and they didn't!

So the first thing to do is sit down and objectively decide if you're playing your own version of this very juvenile and very fattening game.

If you are, that's great, because your course of action is clear: buy snacks *they* like and you don't. If they want cakes and pastries, get some that have fillings that are acceptable to them but not at all appetizing to you. Get flavors of ice cream that bore you or turn you off but that the others can enjoy.

14

Eating Out

Americans are now eating more than one out of every three meals away from home, and the percentage is rising rapidly. That trend poses some very difficult challenges to weight-conscious people. On the other hand, eating at a restaurant can be very enjoyable, and, if you handle it right, an integral part of your reducing or weight-control program.

When I was a kid, the kind of restaurant where I was taken most frequently would typically serve a meal consisting of a small salad, a serving of something like chicken or Salisbury steak, mashed potatoes, a green vegetable, and some kind of dessert, usually nothing more exotic than a small serving of ice cream or pie. A meal like that had a definite rhythm and structure to it and was reasonably well balanced. The design of the menu and even the way the meal was served did not invite either overly rapid eating or overindulgence.

The typical restaurant today is nothing like that. Fast-food establishments are the overwhelming presence almost everywhere you go, and at least two of the big chains are building new establishments at the rate of more than one a day. The average American now eats *nine* meals a month at a fast-food restaurant. You may think that the market is already saturated, but research tells me we haven't seen anything yet.

One of the big troubles with fast-food places is that they *are* fast-food places. You not only get served fast, you eat fast, too. And eating fast is not a good idea for people like you and me. We need to give our stomachs time to realize that we *are* eating. Even worse, many of the foods featured in fast-food establishments have astonishingly large amounts of calories, considering their relatively small satisfaction value. A Big Mac, for instance, has 540 calories. A Whopper really is: 630 calories. A typical *meal* at McDonalds might include a Big Mac, french fries, and a vanilla milk shake. That socks you with 1,074 calories! Add the apple pie dessert and you're up to 1,374 calories.

There also seems to be a trend for fast-food establishments to serve ever-larger amounts of fats and oils. I used to think Arthur Treacher's was bad until I tried another establishment with a seafood theme and discovered the repulsiveness of tiny pieces of shrimp and chicken tucked into thick suitcases of greasy batter.

There are even more insidious trends. The Coca-Cola company has been mounting a big campaign to convince fast-food operators to offer 20-ounce servings as the new "large" size. And the early returns show that many people are in fact buying that size — which contains 240 empty calories, the equivalent of about 16 teaspoons of sugar! In malls, the hottest new trend is shops selling nothing but cookies. Other new operations specialize in deep-fried bread. I don't know what they could follow that act with, except maybe fried candy with whipped cream on top. . . . Anyone for a franchise?

Are there any *good* trends in the fast-food world? Well, I see a few. Some chains are now opening salad bars. If you don't overindulge on the dressings, you can't go too far wrong with the salad bar, even in a fast-food restaurant, although you might gain a few extra ounces by absorbing some of the air-borne grease. In some restaurants, you are invited to order your burger the way you want it, which means that you could order it without fat-laden sauce, but if there are lines in a restaurant, that can be awkward. For that reason, I like what's going on at a chain called Wendy's. There, you *have* to tell them what you want on your hamburger, which means you can order it with lettuce, tomato, onion, and catsup, all of which add a lot of taste but no more than about 20 or 25 calories. Even better, Wendy's sells some very tasty, piping hot chili con carne with beans. It comes with a couple of crackers, and the whole package is good for about 400 calories, I'd estimate. Aside from the fact that I happen to like well-prepared chili and beans, I recommend this because it's more like the food in traditional restaurants. The chili is very hot, so it takes a long time to eat. The beans are filling, and have a lot of fiber, which is all but entirely absent from most fast foods. It's surely just as filling, if not more so, than a Big Mac or a Whopper, yet it has about 140 calories less than a Big Mac and 230 calories less than a Whopper.

The kind of restaurant where you can sit down and enjoy a leisurely meal presents a different kind of challenge. Some people can handle it rather well, others poorly. Until very recently, I was in the latter category. Every time I left a restaurant, my belt seemed to have shrunk at least an inch. The typical scenario for a lunch in those days went something like this:

I'd sit down, look over the menu, and usually decide to order a chef's salad. I like salad, and besides, I thought, "a chef's salad is not fattening." But it usually takes some time to prepare a chef's salad, and frequently, more than one person at my table would order one. Meanwhile . . . *rolls.* Invariably, the waitress would place a wicker basket of rolls, rye bread, and crackers at the table, demurely wrapped in a napkin, along with a big, golden blob of butter. "Well, as long as I'm only having a chef's salad . . . one won't hurt." Of course, there were often *two* rolls, and some crackers as well, but. . . .

Finally the salad would come, complete with a gravy boat full of blue cheese or Roquefort dressing, and the better part of it would be strewn over the salad. And after that? At least half the time, dessert. And as I'd lurch my way toward the door, I'd invariably wonder why or how I managed to make such a pig of myself.

When I began my reducing program, it didn't take long to realize that I was making at least two major errors. First, of course, was eating all those rolls, more out of *impatience* for my real lunch than a desire to eat the rolls. Even in good restaurants, it is extremely rare to get bread that is really worth eating. But I would eat it anyway. The second error, surprisingly enough, was ordering that chef's salad. But let's look at these strategic mistakes one at a time.

Theoretically, a buttered roll before dinner could serve as the protein and fat combination that we suggest for beginning a meal. But for some reason, rolls don't seem to slow down your appetite. At least not mine. About all they do is add empty calories to your meal. If you went for a 30-minute walk to reach the restaurant, the entire caloric benefit of that walk will be wiped out by one buttered roll. Eat two and you've negated the benefit of the walk home. Do you really want to walk one hour for two rolls?

I simply used to tell myself that I wasn't going to eat any rolls, but I would anyway. Finally, I began telling the waitress not to bring rolls, or to take them away if the busboy had brought them. Unfortunately, this technique is only possible when eating by yourself or with a close friend. As an alternative, when there are a number of people at the table, you can simply arrange to have the rolls set beyond arm's reach. If you feel you must *do something* while waiting for your food, drink water and talk like crazy. Think about the real food you're going to get soon, and realize that it is likely to be very filling and satisfying without any help from those rolls.

To tell the truth, it took me at least a year to be able to handle rolls, but I've finally done it. Now, I simply regard them as part of the decor, and I don't think about eating them any more than I would think about eating pieces of wax fruit, which white rolls rather resemble anyway.

The chef's salad fiasco. I am not alone in liking chef's salads — or at least, I wasn't, because I don't eat them anymore. Some people, I suspect, order them in a restaurant as a kind of gesture to others (and maybe even themselves) that they really have small appetites and wouldn't think of eating a big meal. But if you think that a chef's salad is some kind of bargain for a reducer, you are deceiving yourself.

Yesterday I had one of our staff call up a very popular local restaurant where I've often eaten a chef's salad. The cook told us exactly what went into each salad, and then we calculated the approximate calories:

	Calories
3 ounces beef	180
3 ounces turkey	155
3 ounces ham	195
3 ounces cheese	315
1 hard-boiled egg	82
4 ripe olives	38
a few slices of onion	5
lettuce	10
½ tomato	20
Total	1,000

To top your salad, you are given approximately four ounces of salad dressing which is equal to about eight tablespoons. Some people don't use all the dressing, so we are giving values for five as well as eight tablespoons.

	CALORIES		
	1 tablespoon	5 tablespoons	8 tablespoons
Blue cheese	76	380	608
French	66	330	528
Italian	83	415	664
Russian	74	370	592
Thousand Island	80	400	640

Incredible, isn't it? Depending upon how much dressing you use, a chef's salad at this restaurant is going to sock you with anywhere from about 1,250 to 1,650 calories.

Granted, some chef's salads are less generous in their portions of meat, but even so, that would only subtract about 175 calories from the imposing total.

Now, suppose you sit down to the table, decide you're going to have a chef's salad, and since it's "just a salad," you decide that you can afford a buttered roll. And maybe you have a glass of wine or beer as well. And possibly dessert. So your caloric total for a chef's salad dinner can easily top 2,000 calories; which is the total *daily* requirement of many people and *more* than the daily requirement of most women.

Our staff researcher was as shocked by these figures as you probably are (she'd eaten plenty of chef's salads herself!) and she was inspired to draw up the following comparison. Suppose, instead of that chef's salad, you had a regular dinner. Which meal would have fewer calories? Consider:

	Calories
1 cup French onion soup with crackers	115
3 ounces lean broiled T-bone steak	190
baked medium potato with sour cream	140
1 cup green beans	30
1 2-inch biscuit with butter	140
1 large piece lemon meringue pie	355
Total	970

Even *with* the sour cream on the baked potato, even *with* the butter on the biscuit, and even *with* the lemon meringue pie, there are still fewer calories in this meal than in the chef's salad — and before you even put any dressing on it!

Luckily, at about the same time that I was bidding farewell to the chef's salad era of my life, salad bars were becoming popular fixtures in restaurants. And frequently, I have the salad bar as my main course — providing it includes protein sources. My favorite salad bar offers, for protein, garbanzos (chick peas), red beans, hard-boiled egg slices, and cottage cheese. Add to your salad bowl or plate plenty of lettuce, onions, cucumbers, tomatoes, mushrooms, scallions, radishes, and other raw vegetables, and you have a total of between 400 and 600 calories, according to my reckoning.

Now, you have to walk before you can run, so when I first discovered salad bars, I used to drench all that low-calorie goodness with tons of fatty dressing. But after a while, I realized that I didn't need that much dressing and gradually began cutting back on it until I now use about two tablespoons for a large salad. That gives me a calorie total of about 550 to 750, which is well under *half* of what I used to get from a chef's salad. And yet, it's just as filling and much more healthful in the bargain.

Enjoying your meal without regrets. I don't believe that all restaurant eating ought to be approached in the same way. A fast meal at a luncheonette or a routine kind of restaurant meal is one thing. "Going out" to a restaurant — regardless of its prices or menu — is something else.

If you *routinely* eat in restaurants, you owe it to yourself to develop new habits of ordering and eating. After all, a few hundred extra calories a few times a week can translate into a lot of fat power. The first thing you have to avoid, as we mentioned before, is consuming rolls and butter simply out of impatience. After that, pay attention to salad dressing. If you aren't used to eating salad without a lot of dressing on it, gradually reduce the amount until you have it down to one tablespoon. If, after giving it an honest try, you discover you can't enjoy it this way, skip the salad. Just make sure that you get some lightly steamed, green, leafy vegetables at home at least three times a week.

Soup is often not a bad bargain. The hotter you get it, the better, because the longer it will take you to eat it, the more it will occupy you and give you a sense of satisfaction. I would also suggest trying to eat your soup without crackers. Again, begin gradually. For the first week, use one less cracker: the second week, two less. Within a month's time you should be weaned away from them without feeling any sense of loss.

When it comes to the main course, my only advice is to avoid anything deep-fried. In general, the cheaper the restaurant, the more white flour and grease is going to surround your meal. Sandwiches spread generously with mayonnaise are almost as bad. The trick, here, I think, is to order foods that you can really *enjoy* without a lot of oil or mayonnaise. Broiled or baked fish is hard to beat for good taste, high nutrition, and low calories. Baked or broiled chicken is another good choice. If you want a potato, choose baked instead of french fried.

As for dessert, for routine meals I believe the wisest course of action is to skip it. If you really want something, the best choice is probably a small dish of ice cream. But even that may get you into trouble, because most adults who are overweight simply cannot make dessert a *routine* part of their diet unless they skimp on needed nutrients.

The "special" dinner is something else. It's not just eating, but a very enjoyable social occasion. It happens anywhere from once a week to once every few months. And the rules are different.

My advice is simply to eat whatever you want. *As long as you really want it.* What I mean is, don't order something just because it looks good on the menu. Or because the waiter has placed it on the table. Instead, study the entire menu, from beginning to end: soup, appetizer, entrée, salad, dessert, and beverage. Create a picture in your mind of a complete meal, and then ask yourself if you really, honestly want any particular component which has attracted your attention. Remember that besides what you see on the menu, there will be bread on the table, too. Imagine how you will feel after eating a roll, an appetizer, an entire platter of food, a salad, dessert, and perhaps wine or coffee. Really imagine it. Will you feel pleasantly satisfied . . . or almost painfully stuffed?

Do you really want that appetizer, or does it just sound cute? Do you really want dessert? If you do, which one? Are you going to have room for it when you are done with your meal? If not, *make* room for it. If you have a choice between a baked potato and french fries, maybe *your* choice will be no potatoes at all. Maybe you'd prefer to order a second green vegetable instead.

Remember that there are more options than you may think. If you want wine, for instance, you don't have to order a full bottle. You may order only half a carafe, which more than likely will be sufficient. Or you can order a single glass of wine. You can order many dishes without the rich sauces they are ordinarily served with. You can have your baked potato without sour cream. You can tell the waiter to use only half the usual amount of dressing on your salad if it is brought to the table already dressed.

The idea, again, is to eat exactly what you want, but *only* what you want. You may well find, as I have, that this more rational way of eating in restaurants not only saves you unnecessary calories, but actually permits you to enjoy your food more, because you have ordered it more carefully, and you feel much more comfortable when it's time to leave.

15

Safeguarding Your Nutritional Health

Many physicians and nutritionists are of the opinion that nutritional supplements are rarely needed, even when you're dieting. The exception to that rule, they'd say, would be people on severe, medically supervised diets, including fasts and modified fasts.

And, on the face of it, the Prevention System of Natural Weight Control is certainly not the kind of diet that produces deficiencies, depending as it does for success on restricting empty-calorie snacks, limiting second helpings, and getting additional exercise. Theoretically, then, there is no need for you to take nutritional supplements.

Unfortunately — or maybe fortunately — we human beings do not live in the neat world of theory but the hurly-burly of reality. So the truth is that although you may not need nutritional supplements in theory, you probably *do* need them in reality. Let me explain why.

First, the fact that you are now embarking on a reduction program suggests to me that in all likelihood you have previously followed a number of other programs, some of them crash diets. Many people, I found, have crash-dieted over and over again.

If that is the case, there is a very good chance that at this very moment you are still suffering from a depletion of nutrients, even though you may not be aware of it. You may even be suffering from health problems associated with those deficiencies — even though neither you nor your physician may link them with your present or past.

Perhaps you have followed numerous diets which produced a

more reasonable weight loss, but still depended for their success on severely restricting your intake of a number of nutrient-rich foods such as milk, cheese, meat, potatoes, and so forth.

If you have a history of dieting, whether it be crash dieting or semicrash dieting, there is an especially high probability that you left yourself with dangerously low reserves of calcium and magnesium. And, if you are a woman, iron.

While most vitamin deficiencies can be compensated for after you go off a diet much more easily than mineral deficiencies, there is still a good chance that your history of dieting has left you with vitamin deficiencies. It's my impression that many dieters become dangerously depleted in B-complex factors particularly, by concentrating on fruits and vegetables while going very light on meat and totally avoiding "starchy" foods such as bread, spaghetti, rice, potatoes, and beans. If milk, cheese, and other dairy products have also been restricted, a B-complex deficiency becomes almost a certainty.

If, after one or more bouts of fairly severe and prolonged dieting, you noticed the development of any one or more of the following conditions, there is a good chance that they came about as a result of poor diet.

- Aching bones or joints — a likely result of calcium deficiency.
- Irritability, difficulty in sleeping, and generally poor nerves — can be produced by a calcium and/or B-complex deficiency.
- Unusually severe menstrual cramps — another possible result of calcium and/or B-complex deficiency.
- Fatigue — can be produced by any combination of deficiencies of magnesium, iron, and B complex.
- Dry, rough, or bumpy skin — a sign of vitamin A deficiency.
- Eczema or other skin rashes — possibly a sign of deficiency of zinc and/or B complex.
- Slow healing following surgery or serious illness — in the dieter, most likely caused by deficiency of protein and zinc, although vitamins A and C are also crucial in healing.
- Constipation — when chronic, usually caused by a deficiency of dietary fiber, particularly fiber from "starchy" foods like bread, beans, and potatoes.

That was just a quick overview, of course, but it is sufficient to suggest that repeated dieting can leave you with health problems that linger — *even after the weight comes back*!

There are other reasons why you may need extra nutritional input besides having a history of dieting. One is that the average American consumes between 20 and 25 percent of all his calories from one single food — sugar. Not natural sugar found in fruits, but sucrose, corn sweeteners, and other refined sugars which are added to thousands of processed foods and which individuals themselves toss into coffee and homemade cakes. That means that 20 to 25 percent of the typical diet is totally bereft of vitamins, minerals, fiber, and other protective elements.

But that's not all. Many Americans take in another 10 percent or so of their total calories in the form of alcohol — beer, wine, or liquor. And as if that weren't bad enough, still more calories are taken in as fat and oils — not the fats and oils found naturally in dairy products, grains, and lean meats — but fats and oils added to processed foods like desserts to give them a richer taste, fat added to hot dogs, sausages, and other cold cuts, fat in which french fries, potato chips, and doughnuts are fried, and the extraordinary amount of saturated fat which occurs in the meat of livestock raised under artificial conditions.

In other words, *one-half or more of the total caloric intake of the average adult American comes from refined sugar, alcohol, and unnatural fat* — substances which humankind did not eat at all until the most recent fraction of a percent of our existence on earth, and which give us no vitamins, minerals, or fiber whatsoever.

Even if you are currently on a weight-reduction program, it's very unlikely that you're going to be cutting out *all* those empty calories. In any case, your past diet probably left precious little opportunity for you to fill your nutritional needs adequately.

Another reason why I feel that many people require nutritional supplementation — and why so many people feel better and become healthier after they supplement their diets — is that most of us today are so sedentary that the total number of calories we consume is much smaller than the amount which nearly everyone ate until the last hundred years or so. A person who does manual labor probably eats between 3,500 and 5,000 calories a day in order to keep his weight steady. Therefore, even if such a person takes in half his calories in the form of sugar, alcohol, and fat, he still has about 2,000 calories left from which to get his vital nutrients.

A typical sedentary adult, on the other hand, may require less than 2,000 — perhaps as few as 1,200 to 1,500 — calories to keep his or her weight steady. Subtract half of that for empty calories and there's very little room for nutritional error.

It is a curious fact of physiology that in general a very active person needs only a slightly greater amount of vitamins and minerals to keep healthy than the sedentary person (a substantial part of the additional need coming from losses through perspiration). The result is that the bookkeeper requires almost as much nutrition as a ditchdigger (except for calories) but is forced to get that nourishment from half as much food. Unless that bookkeeper's food selections are very wise indeed, he or she stands a fairly high risk of walking around with very low nutritional reserves, if not of suffering from an outright deficiency problem.

But then what happens when that bookkeeper diets repeatedly over a period of years? The risk, common sense tells us, escalates from fairly high to very high.

To change our perspective from one of different occupational patterns to individual eating habits, I have noticed that many dieters substantially increase their intake of coffee. They do this for a number of reasons, including putting something warm in their mouths that has no calories and getting a boost from the caffeine. But what few coffee hounds realize is that when you begin drinking more than a couple of cups of coffee (or tea) a day, you begin to destroy a B vitamin called thiamine. Thiamine is especially important for your mental and psychological health. So the person who cuts back on his food intake while increasing his coffee intake is putting himself at a double risk of developing nervous problems because of a vitamin deficiency.

Still another reason is that, even when they are following a perfectly sensible diet, many people simply can't help but overdo it. They begin skipping meals, cutting normal portions of meat and chicken in half, avoiding bread, beans, and potatoes completely, practically living on toast, cottage cheese, grapefruit, and coffee. Yet, if you ask them, they will say they're following a sensible diet suggested by their doctor. But just as surely as the person who freely admits he is on an out-and-out crash diet or even a fast, the person overdoing that basically reasonable diet is headed for multiple deficiencies and multiple health problems.

Finally, I suggest that most dieters would be better off with supplementation for the simple reason that most dieters are women.

And most women do not get nearly enough calcium — even when they *aren't* dieting — with the result that they are at high risk of developing any one or more of a number of problems associated with calcium deficiency. These include osteoporosis, or a thinning of the bones, often accompanied by pain; cramps or muscle spasms, particularly in the legs; nervousness, irritability, and insomnia; even dental or gum problems, produced by the receding of the bony crest which holds the teeth in place. What's more, although calcium deficiency is definitely not recognized by the majority of doctors as a contributing factor in arthritis, it is my overwhelming impression that in *some* cases, it is.

Having said all that, let me admit that many health professionals would not agree that most women are in need of more calcium. Some *would*, though — and by no coincidence — because they are the doctors who have actually studied calcium metabolism in large groups of women, using the latest research tools and a variety of approaches to the problem. The consensus among these researchers is that calcium deficiency may very well be (it's impossible to prove this sort of thing absolutely) a major contributing factor to health problems in older women.

One revealing study published by three M.D.'s at the Creighton University School of Medicine in Omaha, Nebraska, late in 1977, suggests that the average woman is getting only about *half* the amount of calcium she absolutely needs. And many women aren't even getting that much! Specifically, these doctors say that the average early-middle-aged woman is actually losing calcium from her bones every day. And they found that to be true even in many women who were eating the "Recommended Dietary Allowance" of calcium for women, which is 800 milligrams a day. Based on the many tests and measurements they performed, these doctors came to the conclusion that the very least amount of calcium that the average woman should be eating to protect herself from this bone-destroying calcium loss is about 1,200 milligrams a day — or half again as much as the RDA. But because that's an average figure, they caution, half of all women will actually need even more than that amount — about 1,500 milligrams a day — simply to balance the calcium that everyone excretes each day as part of the body wastes. (For fuller details of this study, including a discussion of how this strange situation has come to exist, see "Calcium Balance and Calcium Requirements in Middle-aged Women" by Heaney, Recker, and Saville, *American Journal of Clinical Nutrition*, October 1977, pp. 1603–11.)

Those are the major reasons why it's likely that nutritional supplements may be important to your health. There are other reasons for nutrient shortages that we could discuss at some length but I will only briefly mention a few: smoking, which destroys vitamin C; the use of steroids, which increases the need for vitamin C and calcium; heavy menstruation, which can lead to depletion of iron reserves; and a history of serious injuries or repeated surgery, which can deplete your body of a wide variety of vital nutrients. Multiple pregnancies can also lead to a nutritionally run-down state, particularly with regard to calcium and B vitamins. It's my impression that women who have borne several children and have also repeatedly dieted are prime candidates for serious nutritional problems.

To safeguard — even better, to *improve* — your nutritional health, there are three steps you must take.

First, because you have a limited number of calories with which to meet your nutritional requirements, you should reduce to a minimum any food which provides nothing but calories — in other words, junk food and snacks. Every calorie that you eat from sugar, fat, or alcohol pushes out a calorie which could simultaneously deliver protein, vitamins, and minerals.

Second, your food selections should focus on items that provide the maximum amount of protective nutrients along with their calories. Such foods include whole grains, fruits, vegetables, eggs, sprouts, fish, poultry, and lean meat. They also include so-called "starchy" foods such as potatoes, beans, and bread. Unless you serve these items drenched with butter or sour cream, they are excellent foods whether you are on a diet or not. Their high-fiber content fills you up and does good things for your digestion and elimination. For the satisfaction they give your stomach, and the nourishment they give your whole body, their calorie content is in no way excessive.

When embarking on a reducing program, it is probably not a good idea to embark simultaneously on a program of eating only health food — or radically changing your diet in any way, for that matter. Don't try to exist on a diet of salads, sprouts, fruits, and vegetables if you're used to eating macaroni, pork chops, and steak. Remember, your strategy is to continue eating the basic foods you like, but to approach them in a much more conscious way so that you will be satisfied with less.

The third step to safeguarding and improving your nutrition is to add the insurance of dietary supplements. In this context, we are not talking about the therapeutic use of nutrition, but simply a broad-spectrum preventive approach. For that purpose, your best bet is to rely on supplements which provide the full range of vitamins and minerals. The potency of each nutrient, which will be clearly stated on the bottle, should be at least 100 percent of the RDA. For vitamins C and E, the potency should definitely be higher than the RDA: at least 100 milligrams a day for vitamin C and 100 international units a day for vitamin E. For women, the protective amount of calcium seems to be about 1,000 to 1,200 milligrams daily—in addition to calcium from the daily diet (which averages about 400 to 600 milligrams). Men can get by with several hundred fewer milligrams.

What about protein supplements? Are they necessary or advisable? In general, probably not, but let me say a few words about what has lately become a very controversial issue.

The major difference between protein supplements and vitamin or mineral supplements is that while a small number of tablets can give you your daily requirement of vitamins and minerals, it's necessary to take about 100 or more protein tablets to fulfill your protein requirement. The typical protein tablet contains only about half a gram of protein and most of us ought to be getting about 50 or 60 grams of protein a day. One average chicken thigh will give you about 15 grams of protein; one small mouthful, then, would provide about 2 grams of protein. So unless it is easier for you to take four protein tablets than it is to eat one forkful of chicken, I don't see any advantage to taking the protein tablets (which also contain calories, by the way).

A more reasonable way to supplement the diet with protein is to find a way to work some brewer's yeast or desiccated liver powder into your daily menu. They will give you some extra protein but also an important bonus of vitamins, trace elements, and other protective substances which are barely understood at this time.

Liquid protein is something else again. The idea is to just about stop eating food altogether and live on liquid protein and vitamin-mineral supplements. That program began as a desperate measure by doctors to reduce people who weighed 300 pounds or more, but quickly degenerated into a commercial circus. Thousands of people began living on nothing but protein drinks for months on end. Complications arose and some of these people even died, perhaps from a deficiency of potassium or other minerals. In any case, the whole business is pathetically pointless, because recent studies show that while enormous weight losses were produced by fasting people under medical supervision, the great majority of them gained back every ounce they lost (and often more!) within a few years.

From all the available research I've seen, protein supplements are in general of much greater value to the person trying to gain weight, or keep from losing it, because of injury, surgery, or illness, than they are to the person trying to lose weight.

A number of people have asked me if taking vitamins increases your appetite, or if vitamins themselves contain calories. To the best of my knowledge, the only circumstances under which taking vitamins will increase your appetite is if your poor appetite is the result of poor nutrition — an ironic situation which can sometimes arise with deficiencies of B vitamins, for instance. But what's really going on here is the *normalization* of appetite through vitamins, not a simple increase. If your appetite is not pathologically poor, it will not be affected by taking supplements. And you need have no fear that the vitamin supplements you take contain calories. The only supplements containing calories are some chewable preparations made with sugar. The number of calories per tablet would probably not exceed about half a dozen. Likewise, there are no calories in minerals such as calcium, iron, zinc, and magnesium.

The only supplements you should be cautious about are those which contain relatively large amounts of oil. I would not think it is a good idea to take large numbers of wheat germ oil perles, for instance. You would be better off eating wheat germ. If you take lecithin, I would recommend the granular form, which is much more concentrated in potency than the capsules. Vitamins A and D are often sold in an oil-base preparation, because they are fat-soluble vitamins, but one small capsule a day should take care of your requirements for these vitamins, so the caloric input would be minimal.

The next logical question is whether or not there are any supplements which can *reduce* your appetite. The answer to that one is a cautious *maybe.*

Some nutritionists suggest that certain cases of excessive eating may be a result of a need to obtain nutrients which are not provided by the normal diet. It's possible, then, that taking a broad range of supplements, including such sometimes-hard-to-get minerals as zinc and magnesium, might reduce your need to go "foraging" for these substances in foods.That's sensible, whether the theory is true or not, and it is even more sensible to make sure that your diet includes a variety of natural foods, including whole grain products, green leafy vegetables, fish, and liver. If you find that your desire for extra foods tends to concentrate on dairy products, you might have to rely on supplemental calcium, because many adults find it difficult, if not impossible, to meet their calcium requirements through food alone. That is particularly true of women.

Some foods which may be thought of as supplements, such as bran, alfalfa, and pectin, may reduce your appetite simply by filling you up, if you take them with meals. Aside from whatever effect they have on your appetite, however, high-fiber foods in general have been shown to reduce the digestibility of calories in the body, an important phenomenon which we discussed in the chapter on natural foods.

Finally, there is a possibility that a few tablespoons of brewer's yeast taken each day may tend to normalize your appetite. I don't know of any clinical data yet on this, but brewer's yeast — not other kinds of yeast — is a rich natural source of a newly discovered nutrient called Glucose Tolerance Factor (GTF), which in many people has a tendency to help normalize blood sugar levels and reduce elevated levels of circulating insulin. Since insulin is believed to have a stimulating effect on the appetite, and since abnormally high levels of this hormone are, according to a recent paper from Johns Hopkins University School of Medicine, "a universal accompaniment of obesity," this lowering effect may be beneficial. It is interesting to note that exercise and a high-fiber diet have a similar effect. In all three cases, this appears to be normalization of a complex set of relationships between insulin, blood sugar, and different body tissues. Let me repeat that brewer's yeast is the only variety of yeast which contains plentiful Glucose Tolerance Factor.

16

Exercise Can Do More for You than You Think

There are many reasons why people gain weight, but if I had to give one reason which I thought was more important than any other, it would not be poor eating habits, the proliferation of snack foods, or the disappearance of natural, high-fiber foods from our diet. If there is one overwhelming, single reason why overweight is such a problem, I would say it was lack of exercise.

And if I were asked to give one, single life-style change which would be the most effective way to lose weight, and keep it normalized, it would be to get more exercise.

Understand, it is entirely possible to lose all your extra weight without getting any more exercise than you are now, but you owe it to yourself to at least try to get more exercise, because it will make you lose weight *faster, easier,* and *more healthfully.* Don't worry if you haven't gotten any exercise at all to speak of for the last 20 years. You can work into it slowly, and you can make it as vigorous or as easy as you like. In fact, if you haven't been getting any exercise, I'm going to *insist* that you make it easy on yourself, very easy, until your body adapts to your new habits.

Why is exercise so important? The obvious answer is that it burns calories. That was the one benefit which everyone in our diet workshop named. A few people named a second reason: it makes you feel better. In reality, there are at least *nine* specific benefits that the weight-reducer can obtain from exercise, and each of them is tremendously important. The fact that so few people appreciate the *depth* of the benefits from exercise is probably one reason why so many simply choose to ignore it.

Before I tell you what these nine benefits are, and how you can put them to work for you, let me take a few minutes to say something about exercise in general, because unless I do, you may think I'm exaggerating when I get down to specifics. What I want to say is that exercise is supremely important for one basic reason: it's *natural.* We human beings are physically put together with muscles capable of extraordinary exertion, and with the capability of putting out work for hours on end. The people who made up the thousands of generations preceding ours made good use of these muscles and this stamina. When you consider the construction of the pyramids, the building of Rome and all the cathedrals of Europe, all of history's herdsmen, farmers, smithies, and foot soldiers, and come right through the ages to our own grandparents and great-grandparents who cracked coal and busted sod for 10 or 12 hours a day, six days a week, you can imagine that all the salt water in the world's oceans could well be humanity's collective sweat.

From the first day that man was created or evolved until the present day, our muscles have enabled us to do the work we *had* to do in order to survive. But in the course of all those hundreds of thousands, perhaps even millions of years, *the relationship between our muscles and our bodies as a whole became one of mutual help and adaptation.* Because our muscles were used so frequently and so strenuously, we developed the ability to provide them with fuel by breaking down carbohydrate, fat, or even protein. We developed efficient ways of providing this fuel on a short-term basis for quick bursts of energy and efficient ways of providing it for marathon feats of endurance. We developed ways of delivering larger amounts of blood to muscles when they need it, and ways of cooling overheated muscles. We developed the ability to make our muscles grow larger and stronger if they were chronically being taxed past the point of their work limits. Our nervous systems developed the ability to program complicated movements into our muscles so that they could carry out difficult tasks without having to get fresh instructions from our conscious minds every instant.

But while all that was going on, there were parallel developments which have enormous consequences for people living in the age of automation. We adapted so well to strenuous, regular exercise that we actually came to *depend* on it. I mean that literally. *Now that we have learned to survive from day to day with very little physical work, the question is whether we can go on doing so very little physical work and survive from year to year.*

Ironically, lack of exercise is so common today that it's difficult to point to any well-identified group of individuals and blame its problems on life-style. Only the extremes tend to stand out. We know, for instance, that when a person is forced to remain in bed for several weeks, debilitating weakness ensues, with loss of body protein, muscle wastage, loss of calcium from the bones, and a greatly increased danger of blood clots due to poor circulation. At the other end of the spectrum, epidemiologists tell us that people who remain very active into their later years will live to see *more* of those later years than their sedentary counterparts.

But for most of us, the damage caused by lack of exercise is most clearly seen when we reverse it with exercise. Some people have such poor circulation in their limbs that they develop severe cramp-like pains on walking a single block. When they are induced to do therapeutic walking, going as far as they can until they must stop, then resting, then walking again, their circulation increases and their condition — intermittent claudication — often improves dramatically. People with varicose veins also benefit by walking, because the contraction of the muscles pushes the blood up through the veins and reduces pressure inside those vessels. When people with serious low back problems do the right kind of stretching exercises, their problem greatly improves and frequently goes away altogether as long as they continue their exercises. Arthritis often responds well to swimming, yoga, and other gentle forms of exercise. Doctors who use walking or jogging as part of a rehabilitation program for heart patients report that it lowers cholesterol, increases high-density lipoproteins in the blood (believed to be protective against heart attacks), improves or abolishes angina, and lowers high blood pressure. Exercise can lower a diabetic's need for supplemental insulin. Psychiatrists are reporting that running greatly improves mood in depressive patients, possibly due to changes in body chemistry. Other doctors use exercise as a natural sedative for patients with sleeping problems. Fewer complications have been reported at childbirth for women who are allowed to walk around freely during the early stages of labor. Migraine headaches are reported to be abolished by jogging in some cases. Muscle tension and other symptoms of anxiety can be made to disappear with exercise. There is some evidence that exercise may be highly protective against gallstones, and animal experiments even suggest that regular exercise can help prevent cancer.

The fact that all these conditions respond well to exercise indicates how basic it is to our well-being. Robert Rodale, the editor of *Prevention* magazine, says that exercise is one of the key components of our "inner historical program," by which he means all those circumstances and activities to which we have adapted during our long history.

Fish gotta swim, birds gotta fly, and we human beings . . . well, we gotta do *something*!

So you see, although exercise may seem alien to you in your present sedentary life-style, your need for this wonderful friend is an important part of your heritage as a human being. And it's high time that you claimed that heritage!

Light your fire. Many of the more troublesome problems that we run across in life cannot be solved simply by direct personal action. There always seem to be complicating factors, like spouses, friends, enemies, money, conscience, and time. Your eating problem is certainly one of the stickier sort, but how encouraging, how motivating it is, to realize that the mess created by that problem can literally be burned away, entirely on your own initiative and say-so! How wonderful if all chronic problems could be dealt with so directly and efficiently!

True, no matter how much exercise you get, you can't burn up your fat in a kind of bonfire; the process is more like applying the small flame of a craftsman's blowtorch. But that's actually good, not bad, because the faster weight goes off, the faster it comes back. And the slower it goes off, maybe, the slower it comes back. That may be even more true for weight loss through exercise than through dieting. In an important study of the effect of walking alone, in which women lost weight at the rate of about half a pound a week, Grant Gwinup, M.D., noted that "Once a certain amount of exercise had produced a certain amount of weight loss, *that loss tended to be maintained with little tendency for a noticeable amount of weight to be regained.*" (*Archives of Internal Medicine,* May 1975, pp. 676–80.)

The second important benefit or advantage of exercise is that *you do not have to eat less in order to lose weight.* It helps, of course, but it isn't a necessity. Those women mentioned before who lost weight through walking alone were told not to change their diets at all during the exercise period. In fact, most of them actually ate *more* than they did before, but they still lost weight. Although the calories burned by the most common forms of exercise do not seem exactly awesome, the cumulative effect over a period of months does — *even more awesome than the cumulative effect of overeating.*

To illustrate this, imagine that you've been gaining weight lately, and put on about 6 pounds in the last year. By continuing to eat the way you have been, you could expect to put on half a pound in the next month. But suppose you began to walk an hour a day, *while continuing to eat just as you were before.* The effect of the walking would ordinarily be enough to cause you to lose about 3 pounds in a month, but even with the excessive eating you continue to do, you would *still* lose 2½ pounds.

I don't necessarily recommend exercising by itself as the best means to lose weight, because most of us find it isn't terribly difficult to cut a few hundred calories out of our daily diets without feeling deprived. But to the extent that reducing your food intake is difficult for you, exercise represents an easy way to reach your goal just the same. It's possible that the problem you have with your eating is of such psychological magnitude as not to respond very well to the principles in this book, or even the ministrations of a therapist. For you, especially, more exercise is the path of least resistance. And if you are substantially overweight, as presumably you are with the kind of problem you have, it's important to know that the heavier you are, the more calories you burn during any given unit of exercise. If you're a 200-pounder and spend an hour walking, you'll be burning up 350 calories, while your 125-pound friend walking along with you will only be burning 235 calories over the same time and distance.

Not having to eat less means that, besides not having to cope directly with your eating problem, you are also avoiding any possible problems that may arise from getting insufficient nutrition on a restricted diet. If you *are* changing your eating habits, as I hope you are, it means that you need only reduce your calorie intake by a very moderate amount to achieve good reducing results.

You may be thinking that for *you,* it would be easier to cut back on calories than to get more exercise, but don't give up yet. Don't even think about it! Later on, I'll give you some tips about how to get started with your exercise program, but right now, let's continue ticking off the benefits to be gained by becoming a more active person.

Change your mind . . . and your body. Anything that makes you *feel* good is good for your reducing program. And nothing I know of makes you feel better longer, and deeper, than exercise. Whether it's a 45-minute stroll through the park, half an hour of jogging, a hike in the mountains, or an hour of handball, exercise seems to make every neuron in your body purr with self-satisfaction. And the older you are, the better it feels. There is a warmth, a deep relaxation and letting-go that comes on you after exercise that makes you feel better all day and sleep better at night.

That's not poetry I'm spouting, but real fact. Blood tests show that prolonged exercise increases the production of certain substances which act as *natural antidepressants.* Other tests show that moderate but regular exercise reduces muscle tension. Ever wonder why you feel so good after an hour of square dancing or splashing around in the surf? It's not just psychological — rather, the classic interface of psychology and physiology.

It's nice to feel good all the time, but it's especially important when you're working on a major project — like losing weight. Anything that makes you feel jittery, anxious, uneasy, dissatisfied, or depressed will make it that much harder for you to focus your attention on what you're doing. Exercise helps you make it easier on yourself.

Another good psychological posture during weight loss is to be actively engaged in a hobby. If you don't have one that's hot at the moment, exercise can fill the bill very nicely. Taking up tennis not only gives you something to do, but something to think about when you aren't doing it. And not only does it fill your mind with images of yourself practicing the basic moves, but those images are of *an active you,* the best kind kind of you there is. A hobby like tennis or skiing or rock hounding also gives you equipment to buy, repair, and worry about. Books to read. New people to meet. Trips to make. It gives your leisure time a definite sense of meaning, of momentum. It keeps you from getting into a situation where life consists of (*a*) working, and (*b*) avoiding the refrigerator.

If your exercise is walking around the neighborhood, that can be a hobby too. I recently bought a soft-cover tree-identification book, and I try to remember to stuff it into my pocket whenever I go for a ramble. I collect leaves and try to make more positive identifications when I return to my home. Another good idea would be to pay close attention to landscaping — assuming there is any in your neighborhood. If not, try to head for the nearest park. Parks were made for walking, after all, and as a taxpayer, why not get your money's worth? Make friends with the trees there and learn their names. Isn't it high time you were an expert in *something*?

Doing your own landscaping is also a perfect combination of exercise with a hobby. Rock gardens, flower beds, stone walkways, and fences all invite your loving attention and sweat. Vegetable gardens are a wonderful exercise-hobby, too. And with gardening, you get the bonus of fresh, low-calorie, high-fiber food. Be sure to plant the rows far enough apart so that you can easily get in between them and weed. The right way to weed, by the way, if you're concerned about physical conditioning, is neither to bend over from the waist nor to squat. Rather, stand back a couple of feet from the weed, and advance one foot so that the outside of your heel is immediately adjacent to the doomed plant. Bend your knees and fall into a deep fencer's stance. Then lean forward just slightly, *keeping your back straight,* grasp the weed firmly with your gloved hand, and yank it smartly out of the ground. Stand up, let your arm fly over your head and hurl the weed out of your garden. Find your next victim close to the row along the other foot and repeat, bending on your other leg. This exercise loosens up your hamstring muscles, strengthens the large thigh muscles, and positively does wonders for your lower back. Throwing the weed away also keeps your shoulders loose. Each cycle, I'd estimate, is good for burning up one solid calorie. Maybe two. The more weeds that grow in your garden, the faster you'll lose weight. That same lunging type of motion, done slowly of course, is also a wonderful way to plant your seeds. If anyone asks you what you're growing in your garden next year, say slender.

The fifth benefit of exercise to the reducer is that when you lose a pound as a result of physical exertion, virtually all the weight you say goodbye to is nothing but fat. But when you lose the same pound through dieting alone, you are bidding farewell not only to some fat, but anywhere from two to ten ounces of lean tissue as well. A loss of lean tissue means you've lost part of those precious muscles in your legs that you count on to carry you around. The muscles that support your spine and hold in your stomach. Muscles you depend upon for good posture and for holding your head up all day without getting tired. It may even mean a loss of connective tissue, cartilage, and probably some of your bones as well. Have you ever gone on a crash diet and quickly lost 25 pounds or more? Did you feel tired, weak? Protein loss could be a factor.

In the studies I've seen, the amount of lean tissue lost by dieting alone ranges from about 10 percent to as high as 65 percent when the weight loss was produced by total fasting. With exercise, the loss of protein is minimal. In fact, with very vigorous exercise, you may well actually *gain* muscle mass even as you lose weight. When you combine a moderate reduction in calories, which we've suggested here, with exercise, the loss of lean tissue would be quite small, and perhaps nil, if you get enough exercise to create some new muscle tissue.

Torch that fat. During prolonged periods of starvation or strict dieting, the body is able to break down protein, play around with its molecules, and come up with fuel that the muscles can burn. But ordinarily, it relies almost exclusively for fuel, on carbohydrates first, and fats second. And that second is a very distant second indeed. Chemically, carbohydrates are *ready* fuel, which can be quickly utilized for energy. Fat, even though it is a much more *concentrated* source of caloric energy, is mostly there as a back-up system and has to be put through considerable engineering before it's ready to be socked into the muscles. If you run down the street to catch your dog, virtually all the energy you burned in that effort came from glycogen, a carbohydrate, stored in your muscles. The lard around your middle just lay there and watched.

But when you *really* get into exercise, taking long hikes or playing tennis, or jogging, your body does some wonderful things. It seems to realize that in order to pursue your new life-style, you are going to need a new system of fuel delivery. One thing it does is store more glycogen, that quick-burn fuel, right in your muscles where it will be needed. But much more important for our purposes, *regular, vigorous exercise increases your ability to burn fat, rather than carbohydrate, as fuel.* To put it just a bit more technically, your ability to mobilize and metabolize free fatty acids increases. Even better, this mobilization of fat as fuel in a well-trained person is a round-the-clock phenomenon: experiments with animals reveal that it continues even under anesthesia!

Normally, the metabolism in "fat depots," as scientists call them (we call them bulges), is very sluggish. Increased metabolism in these areas may have something to do with the creation of bigger and better blood vessels in the area, which result from the body's need to send hot blood from exercising muscles up through the fat to the skin, where it can be cooled by exposure to air. In any event, it's clearly a beautiful example of adaptation, with your body changing itself to accommodate your changing needs. And the net result is that if you get into a regular program of vigorous, sweaty activity, those bulges which may have seemed impervious even to your best dieting efforts will begin to shrink noticeably.

The seventh advantage of exercise is that its benefits tend to be progressive. The exercise you do this week will make the exercise you do next week easier — encouraging you to do more. The first time I went jogging, as slowly as I could, I managed about 200 yards before I had to stop and get my breath. Three or four months later I had to run 2 or 3 miles just to feel as though I were warmed up. A year later, I ran 18 miles, up in the mountains, and *never* got out of breath, just energy. So you see, it doesn't matter how poor your ability or endurance is in the beginning. It's a wonderful experience to feel your stamina increasing week by week, and to realize that you can burn away up to 600 calories an hour in the process of making yourself feel good all over.

Advantage number eight of exercise to the reducer is that group of health benefits we discussed earlier. I mean, I want you to live, and to be healthy, so you can *enjoy* your new slenderness! As an overweight person, you see, you are particularly prone to a large number of health problems, and exercise can help abolish or prevent nearly every last one of them. That includes atherosclerosis (clogging of the arteries), high blood pressure, aches in your feet and legs, low back problems, poor endurance, and shortness of breath. Overweight people in their mature years tend to develop diabetes, and exercise is now considered important in the treatment of this increasingly common disease, tending to lower the need for supplemental insulin. Statistically, fat people are even more prone to develop cancer, but at least one experimental study with mice showed that animals who were given vigorous daily exercise had much greater resistance to cancer than animals who did nothing but sit and dream about cheese all day.

Cool your appetite. The final benefit of exercise — that I know of, anyway — is that when you get enough of it, the kind that makes you huff a lot and maybe even puff a little, it depresses your appetite. Yes, *depresses.* The common idea that exercising stimulates your appetite is completely false. It may be true for people who are underweight, but not for people like you and me. What's really happening, I think, is that as exercise normalizes a variety of your body functions, it also normalizes your appetite. It puts you more in touch with yourself, with your true needs, and removes you and your appetite from the grasp of mere habit. Possibly, this appetite-normalizing effect has something to do with a reduction in the circulating levels of insulin, since insulin is believed to stimulate the appetite. And fat people, remember, have abnormally high levels of insulin. It may also have something to do with the fact that the well-conditioned person is burning a greater percentage of fat, rather than carbohydrate, to provide energy. Since fat is such a concentrated source of energy, the body's master control may figure that there's no pressing need for large amounts of food, and accordingly turn down the appetite a notch or two.

The fact that vigorous exercise normalizes appetite has not been convincingly demonstrated in a scientific way, but I know that it had that effect on me, and that many people who've seriously taken up jogging say the same thing. One study with mice, however, did show quite clearly that animals who exercised in a rotating drum actually ate *less* than animals which were not exercised. My own feeling is that when a person who has become much more conscious of eating, as you have, takes up exercise, the probability that he will be able to eat less is very high.

No-sweat exercise. This past summer, I went to a wedding at the home of a woman whom I'll call Mrs. Garber. The first thing I noticed is that she had seemingly gained a good 20 pounds, maybe 30 (strange, isn't it, how extraordinarily sensitive we are to changes of weight — in *other* people!). During the ensuing proceedings, Mrs. Garber certainly didn't stuff herself. In fact, she ate very lightly. Why, then, had she gained so much weight?

For all that we've said about the desirability of vigorous exercise, Mrs. Garber didn't get fat because she failed to take up cross-country skiing. In all likelihood, she became unhealthfully and unattractively overweight because *she stopped getting exercise that she didn't even know she was getting.*

Back in the days when we lived on the same street, Mrs. Garber, like everyone else, walked two blocks a day, just about *every* day, to get to and from the corner grocery store. The row homes we lived in then all sat on a small embankment, and everyone had to walk up a dozen or more concrete steps to reach their front door. Inside each house, the bathroom and all the bedrooms were on the second floor, and the laundry was down in the cellar (we didn't call it a "basement" in those days). Each house had a garage in the rear, and after you parked your car, you had to walk up a steep flight of back steps to reach the rear entrance.

Today, Mrs. Garber lives in a ranch home. Everything is on one level, so she doesn't have to go up and down a flight of stairs every time she visits the bathroom. She doesn't have to go down the stairs and up the stairs carrying a basketful of clothing when she does her laundry. When she parks her car, she doesn't have to climb a steep set of stairs to get into her house; in fact, she may not even have to open her garage door, but simply press a button. Once in the garage, she gains immediate and direct entrance to her home. And, no doubt, she uses her car to do all her shopping nowadays. While she once had to lug packages back from the store, and then up the steps, now she just puts them in the back of her car and that's that.

Now that I think of it, back in the old days, it was common for women to go to a shopping area about five blocks away several times a week, and when they did so, it was almost always on foot. The drugstore that everyone went to was three or four blocks away, the dry-cleaning shop, a block away, and the barber and beauty shop, two blocks. And all of us walked.

If you estimate the additional number of calories that Mrs. Garber was spending back in those days, including all that walking and stair climbing, as well as having far fewer conveniences like automatic washer-dryers to use, you might come up with a figure of about 250 calories a day.

If someone goes on eating the same way they were before, but expends 250 calories less a day in physical activity, they will begin to gain weight and will continue to do so until they have put on nearly 18 pounds of flab. At that point, the caloric cost of carrying around that extra fat will stop the gain. Actually, Mrs. Garber looked as if she had gained more than 18 pounds, but that may well have been a result of poor muscle tone in the abdominal region, causing her belly to protrude. But the point is that it is extremely easy — almost logical, you might say — for someone to put on an extra 20 pounds simply as a result of moving from one place and one style of life to a more "modern" style of living.

Probably, if you are over 40 or 50, that true story about Mrs. Garber will sound very familiar. And so will her weight problem. Yet, you may not have thought of your excess weight as being the result of lack of exercise, because you never considered walking to the grocery store or up and down a flight of stairs to visit the bathroom as "exercise." But it is. It may not give you the body of a Greek goddess, but it sure enough burns calories. And if failing to get that exercise inevitably puts pounds on, getting more of that kind of "invisible" exercise will inevitably take them off.

It would be convenient if we could get rid of some of our conveniences, wouldn't it? Jack up our houses 20 feet in the air so that we had to walk up the steps to reach the front door. And put the bathroom up on the roof. But we can't, any more than we can walk three miles down a suburban road with no sidewalk to reach the supermarket. So what we do is play games. Weight-losing games that use spare moments here and there to bring back some semblance of an earlier and more active life-style.

Do you drive to work? Park your car a couple of blocks away and walk the rest of the way. Instantly, you are back to the days when you (or your parent) walked to the local grocery store. Want to speak to someone while you're at work? Instead of using the telephone, walk to their office. It's like walking down the street to drop in on a neighbor. Break time? Spend it walking; you just went to the neighborhood drugstore. Is there an elevator in your building? Use the stairs instead. Rest between flights if you want to; even half-way up each flight if you have to. But *use* those stairs, just like all of us did years ago.

If you live in a house where there are stairs, consider yourself lucky. A staircase is the best piece of exercise equipment ever invented. Walk up and down, twice, every hour on the hour. Or every time there is a commercial break on TV. If you have more than one phone in the house, send the extra ones back to the phone company. Whenever you find yourself in front of the sink, do half a dozen knee bends and half a dozen toe-raises. Whenever you want to pick something up off the floor, use the same exercise we described for weeding. Talking on the telephone? Stand, don't sit, and do leg raises and semisquats. Use your imagination. Every little movement helps. If it makes you grunt, all the better. Here's your big chance to be a pig.

Walk away from it all. Changing a few little habits here and there is a good way to burn off maybe 50 to 100 calories a day. But in addition to that kind of exercise, you want to make vigorous, honest-to-goodness exercise part of your life-style. It will speed your weight loss, increase the mobilization of fat, make you feel better, and help normalize your body chemistry. The best way for most people to do all that is to get into the habit of taking at least one long daily walk.

Walking is something that requires no special training, coordination, skill, or clothing. Well, it does require a good, comfortable pair of shoes, but that's about all. If you don't have such a pair of shoes, by all means buy one tomorrow. You can't pound nails with a hammer that is three inches long, and you can't walk with a pair of shoes that's too tight. Believe me, it will be the best investment you ever made, because walking *anywhere* is your path to salvation.

Even though I'm a jogging nut myself, I still recommend walking as the best form of exercise because the chances that you're really going to *do* it are much greater. Besides that, many people who jog give up after a few months when they develop knee pain. In fact, I ran into knee pain myself, not once, but several times, and if I didn't love jogging so much, I would have given it up long ago. As it is now, I'm still experimenting with different remedies to try to solve the problem. In the meantime, I've taken up racquetball, but mostly, I'm *walking.*

I've always thought there was something special about walking ever since I read that Charles Dickens, my favorite novelist, used to spend practically all night walking the streets of London, mile after mile. Someone has said that the jogger is looking for something, while the walker has found it.

When I was younger I used to walk a lot because I had to. Now I walk because I have to again — not because I don't have a car, but because I need the exercise. The town I live in, like many towns, has a hiking club, and that's how I got started. Many newspapers now carry schedules of weekend events, and chances are a local hike is on the docket. Usually, these hikes are easy, just enough to get you mildly sweaty, which is the best of all states to be in. But these weekend hikes should serve mainly to stimulate you and give you recreation. Walking once a week isn't nearly enough.

Earlier, I talked about getting started with walking when I was discussing how exercise can become a hobby. But the most important thing of all about walking is actually getting out there the very first time. It is that way with a lot of things in life. Taking the plunge is the hard part; the rest is easy. Objectively, it may not seem like there is anything very daring about simply going for a walk, but I'll be the first to admit that making a change in your daily routine is one of the most difficult things you can do. But it's also one of the most important.

The number of calories that you burn by walking depends on how much you weigh and where you're walking. If you are toddling along at two miles per hour, which is about the speed at which you'd be going past an interesting showcase window, you will be burning about 145 calories an hour if you weight about 120 pounds, 185 calories if you weigh 150, and 215 calories if you weigh 200 pounds. With moderate walking, at three miles an hour, you will burn between 235 and 350 calories per hour, depending on your weight. At four miles an hour, which is brisk walking, the kind you do when you're really serious about getting someplace, the values range between 270 and 400. If you are walking up a grade which is just steep enough to make you bend forward a little in order to balance yourself better, you would be burning up *twice* the number of calories that you would walking on the level. Don't, however, go out hunting hills the very first day. Work up to them slowly. If the weather seems uncomfortably cold for walking, be grateful, because walking in the cold air burns up 7 to 10 percent more calories than walking in balmy June weather — a result of increased metabolic needs to keep yourself warm, and the burden of wearing winter clothing. Extremely hot weather also causes a small increase in caloric expenditure, but I don't recommend it. The best time to take your summer walks is early in the morning, while the sun is still low.

Get fit while you get thin. Walking is the most sensible, realistic form of exercise for most people, but if you have a powerful impulse to get fit while you get thin, and to get thin faster, by all means give in to it and try some vigorous sports.

You say you're not interested in sports? That you can't imagine yourself jogging in your wildest dreams? That you don't have time for an exercise program? That's exactly what *I* said not long ago to a physical fitness and life-style coach named Dyveke Spino. I was visiting Dyveke (pronounced Duŕ-vick-a) at her home base in Mill Valley, California, as part of a journalistic investigation of holistic health trends in California. But Dyveke insisted she didn't want to be just interviewed; she wanted me to get actually involved in her program.

"Listen, Dyveke, I'm a very busy person. I'm the editor of a magazine. I write books. I travel a lot. I mean, I just don't have the time to get involved in a serious exercise program. Besides, you're going to tell me to jog, aren't you? I tried that once, when I used to belong to the Y; I used to jog around the inside track and it was the most boring thing I ever did in my whole life. So let's just get on with the interview, huh?"

Dyveke had heard it all a hundred times before. She gently led me through about 10 minutes of self-exploration, in which I examined my daily schedule, mentally rearranging things in an attempt to free up some time. We finally decided that since I wasn't doing anything too earth-shaking during the hour or so before I went to bed, I would try retiring earlier, then arising earlier, so that I would have a solid hour to spend on exercise while I was still fresh.

"But you see, where I live, out in the country, you can't jog along the roads, because they wind all over the place and there's no shoulders. It's very hilly, too, and the cars can't see you until they're right on top of you."

"Well, what about parks?" Dyveke asked. "Fields, playgrounds?"

There are plenty of those, I had to admit. But they were a ten-minute drive away.

So I drove. By the dawn's early (or late) light, I began jogging around a dew-covered ball field. Ten minutes to get there, ten minutes of jogging, ten minutes to get home, and I had an exercise program. As the weeks passed, the ten minutes in the middle began to grow steadily. After about two months, I switched to another park, which runs along a small river, and before too long I was putting in four to five miles of jogging a day without any great strain, and my whole program was only taking up one hour, which didn't interfere with any of my other activities.

The point is, you have more time than you think you do. All you have to do is look for it, *really* look for it, and you'll find it. Don't think of your schedule in such broad terms as working, cooking, doing housework, and then going to bed. Get yourself a nice big tablet, actually write down what you do hour by hour, 24 hours a day. Then do a little engineering, a little juggling, and see what you can come up with. If you're married, by all means take your spouse and even your children into consideration. Maybe they would like to do something with you, or perhaps you can induce them at least to try. How about swimming at the Y, tennis, folk dancing, jogging, handball, racquetball, karate, Tai-Chi, ice skating, volleyball or badminton?

If you find your schedule somehow resistant to your best efforts, or if you haven't even bothered to write out your schedule, I want you to think about the following question, and give it a very serious answer: *What is the significance of the fact that you seem to have no time in your schedule to call your own?* To devote to your own precious health and recreation? Think about it. Is that a very wise lifestyle? Or even reasonable?

Many women seem to feel that they'd somehow be "cheating" their husbands or their children by "selfishly" taking an hour of their time to devote to exercise. If that is your case, please take the time to think about another question: *Are you doing your husband or your children any kind of favor by wearing yourself out?* By not improving your health and appearance? Do you think they love you more because you spend every available minute at their service or in their company? Finally, ask yourself if it's possible, just possible, that by taking the time to exercise, to become fit, to become more slender, you might actually be improving your relationship with your family. No, it won't happen the first week, not usually. Men sometimes become childishly resentful and cranky when their wives begin to take time for themselves. Your kids may even laugh at you. But that won't last long, believe me.

Barbara worked on herself mentally for at least two months before she was able to get it all together and begin her jogging program. After all her work, including the techniques of Super-Positive Thinking, which we describe later, she donned her sweat suit and hit the road. Her husband greeted this effort with nothing but derisive laughter. Laughter gave way to mocking, and finally he even accused her of inviting the lustful stares of strange men, perhaps even a sexual attack. But Barbara persisted, never arguing with her husband, or making counterremarks. Six weeks later, her husband suddenly announced *he* was going to begin jogging, too. Now he enjoys it more than she does, and never misses a day.

Some women don't need men to discourage them. They do it themselves, most frequently by imagining that they'll look foolish jogging or playing tennis or swimming. They imagine that everyone is going to stare at them and think lewd thoughts. The first thing I want to say about that fear is that men, anyway, do *not* think that women engaged in sports look either stupid or sexually brazen. Do you know what they *do* think? Nothing. They simply couldn't care less. The second thing I want to say is that the foregoing should properly be of no consequence: what in the world do you care what other people — whom you don't even know — think when they see you exercise? Do you raise your children the way you think other people would like you to? Read books or watch TV programs that you think other people would endorse?

Realize, then, that any doubts or hesitations you have are your very own private doubts and hesitations. And in a way, they're perfectly legitimate — to a point. Sure, we kind of laugh at ourselves when we start doing something we aren't familiar with — whether it's exercising or enrolling in an evening course. It's a kind of nervous laughter, though, that quickly evaporates, often in a matter of minutes.

Choose a form of exercise that you think you'll enjoy. If you can't think of a particular one, then think of a *place* that you'd like to be. Do you like the park? Then that's the place for you. Do you like the ambience of the tennis court? A swimming pool? Go there, and start batting a ball around or getting your feet wet. If, after all I've said, you still feel a little embarrassed about jogging around your neighborhood, then drive to some other neighborhood, and jog there. In fact, I did something like that myself. As I mentioned before, I had previously jogged on an inside track at the Y. I found it not only boring, but extremely noisy and much too hot. By shifting my place of exercise to a nearly empty athletic field, I could enjoy the grass, the trees, a soft running surface, perfect quiet, and the cool, fresh, morning air.

Whatever you decide to do, start slowly. Very slowly. Almost ridiculously slow. You see, your muscles may not ache the first few times you're out doing your thing, but a few days later, the pain will catch up with you, and if you've overextended yourself, you may be sore for three or four days. So do *less* than you can. Make it easy on yourself. The first few weeks, progress will be slow, but as you very gradually advance, you will discover that your body is making some wonderful adaptations, and that you can do a lot more with less strain. Best of all, what seemed like torture the first week will actually become pleasurable by the beginning of the second month, and absolutely exhilarating by the third month. Every system, physical and mental, will be adapting to your new life-style. You will be absolutely astonished at how much more endurance your muscles have. Your wind will become almost inexhaustible. Cramps, aches, and side stitches will become a thing of the past.

I never cease to be amazed at the way the body changes to accommodate us. When I first began to jog, I was surprised that I perspired very little. My clothing would be damp when I was running, but that's about all. About two months later, while jogging, I suddenly became aware that I was sweating freely. Yet, I had only run about two miles, which was not a greater distance than I had run before without sweating. For a long time, I couldn't understand why that was so. Why hadn't I sweated before, when I was carrying more fat, and running was a much greater effort? I found out the answer to that one just yesterday, when I read a report by scientists who showed that well-trained runners begin to perspire much earlier in a race than others. Why? Apparently, it's an adaptation that serves to cool off the well-conditioned athlete right from the beginning of his exertions, helping to prevent dangerous overheating even after hours of vigorous exercise. How's that for being accommodating? Thanks, body.

If you do your exercise at the Y or at a country club, you will see a lot of people slaking their thirst on the likes of Coke and beer. And hear them complaining about how difficult it is for them to lose weight. They might as well be drinking pure fat. Learn to slake *your* thirst on water. Water gets your thirst better than any other beverage, and gives you that deep down clean feeling. Don't be afraid to drink all you want. No matter how much you consume, you won't gain an ounce — except until the next time you go to the bathroom. Vigorous athletics can make you lose more water than you think, so be sure to replace it, taking frequent drinks throughout the day. Be sure not to misinterpret thirstiness at night for hunger.

You'll notice that as your exercise program continues, and you lose weight, your performance will almost automatically improve. And that will give you good motivation to keep losing. Sports and weight control make beautiful partners.

17

The Technique of Super-Positive Thinking

What you're doing isn't exactly easy. If you haven't admitted it yet, admit it now.

We humans are remarkably adaptive in the face of adversity or coercion. Although a few seem unable to cope with the stress, the great majority of us manage to do very well when it comes to surviving changes of habit imposed upon us by shortages, upheavals, or catastrophes. When food becomes too expensive or scarce, we learn to plant gardens. When gasoline becomes hard to get at any price, we learn to form car pools. When storms damage our property, we make repairs. When we move, we make new friends. We lose a job and find another. And in all but the worst cases, new patterns of living soon replace the old ones. Unless what was lost gave immeasurable meaning to one's existence — like a loved one — life doesn't seem any the worse — or any different, really — under the new regime.

It's a different story, though, when we aren't being *forced* to change. Many of us have an incredibly difficult time changing habits which add no meaning or fun or love whatsoever to our lives. Whether it's eating binges or smoking incessantly or not getting any exercise, changing is a lot easier said than done. Why? Well, I suppose that's what's meant by "force of habit." And it's a force that you'll be confronting and skirmishing with time and time again as you carry out your weight-loss program.

When you're changing a habit, you can be influenced to a

considerable degree by your environment. If you were trying to give up cigarettes, for instance, and you got a new job in an office where nearly everyone smoked, you would deserve a medal if you were able to carry out your plan to quit successfully. But if you were to get a new job where almost no one smoked, where smoking was prohibited in certain areas, and where several co-workers were allergic to smoke, your environment would be giving you no less than three different messages that smoking is socially unacceptable and that not smoking is the normal thing to do.

I don't know what kind of total environment you live in, but one environment that about nine out of ten people live in is the world of television. If you watch as much as the average person, you are getting zapped every day of your life by a constant barrage of suggestions to eat, eat, eat. And I think I'm safe in saying that no less than 80 to 90 percent of food or beverage ads on TV are for junk foods and junk beverages. Soda. Beer. Candy and mints. Corn chips and cheese crackers. Potato chips and chocolate chip cookies.

The more sugar, grease, or salt there is in a food, the more money is spent advertising it on TV.

Perhaps you're thinking, that may be so, but I don't listen to those ads. Well, maybe you don't, but that laboratory mouse inside you, the one we talked about before, has his pink little ears turned up and his nose is twitching away like mad. Your subconscious is getting a message that junk food is fun food. And even if you never act upon that insidious message being pumped into your ears by Madison Avenue, the mere fact that these images are stored in your cerebral cortex can give you problems. It tends to add force to phony eating impulses and increase the sense of uneasiness that may arise when you are learning to eat in a more discriminating manner.

I'm not trying to discourage you or frighten you. But these two factors — the force of habit and the junk food mantra of TV advertising — may be causing you problems right now. Your program may be going along pretty much the way you would like it to, but it may seem like it's draining a lot of your energy. And with two big negatives like old habits and images of food advertising working against you, it's no wonder that losing weight is no lark.

Fortunately, there is a very effective way of making your new program of sensible eating a lot easier.

It's properly known as self-hypnosis or autosuggestion, although I prefer to think of it as Super-Positive Thinking. It's no miracle, and certainly no substitute for consciously changing your eating behavior. But it helps. Exactly how much is hard to say because it will vary greatly from person to person. Looking back, I'd estimate that using autosuggestion increased the effectiveness of my weight-reducing program by about 20 percent. But a woman I know said she simply couldn't get started at all until she used it. Then everything fell into place and her reducing program was off and running.

Experience has taught me that many people are very suspicious of self-hypnosis, no matter what name you give it. They picture hypnosis as a deep, mysterious trance associated with conniving men with bushy eyebrows, or old-fashioned stage entertainers. When I told one of our workshop classes that I was going to introduce them to self-hypnosis in the next session, not everyone was enthusiastic. One person told me he was afraid he wouldn't be able to "come out of it." Another person told me she was against it on religious grounds — explaining that her faith regarded hypnosis as a turning inward, whereas the right direction to look was toward the universe, to God.

Since I gave up arguing about religion during my first year of college, I didn't suggest to this woman that God may be inside us just as he is outside us. In fact, I said nothing at all except that I would understand why she wouldn't be at the next workshop. Hypnosis *is* a kind of touchy subject and it's my policy never to persuade anyone to try it unless they really want to. And of course, that goes for you, too.

But let me hasten to add that experience has also taught me that many people don't really know what self-hypnosis is all about. It would be a shame for these people not to get to know a little more about it before rejecting it out of hand. I say that because not long ago, I was one of those people.

What is self-hypnosis? Self-hypnosis, the kind I'm going to teach you to do, does not induce what you would ordinarily consider a "deep trance." It does not make you feel spacey or dizzy. Self-hypnosis is basically a form of deep relaxation, and that is how you will feel. Not sleepy-relaxed, but relaxed and alert. Above all else, you feel *comfortably relaxed.*

The sensation of being under self-hypnosis is in reality so *un*-strange that we sometimes have to do little tricks to help convince ourselves that we are in fact in a state of altered consciousness.

Another fear you can dispose of is that you "won't be able to come out of it." That simply cannot happen. The altered state of awareness you find yourself in under self-hypnosis is so fragile, really, that there's almost nothing *to* come out of. If some kind of household emergency were to arise while you were doing self-hypnosis, you would be able to break out of it instantly, quite as easily or even more easily than if you had been dozing off while watching TV.

But isn't hypnosis a kind of self-deception? you may be thinking. Isn't it a gimmick? And how can it be called *natural?*

Those are all good questions.

When we practice self-hypnosis, what we are doing is energizing our bodies, our reflexes, and our behavior with the desires of the most rational part of our brains.

We've already seen how so much of our behavior is controlled by habits, causing us to perform many rituals without really being aware of what we are doing. Think of those habits, those conditioned responses, as *negatives* which have become deeply ingrained in our nervous systems.

We also know that our environment may be giving us subtle but powerful messages that reinforce these negatives. There are the thousands of junk food ads on TV, the displays in the pastry shop window, the candy bars next to the check-out counter at the supermarket. There are the friends and possibly family members who are always pushing food in your direction, and always the wrong kind of food. Food processing and packaging, which makes junk foods artificially attractive, are also powerful but often unrecognized negatives.

As if all that weren't bad enough, you may even be in a situation where certain people are telling you that there's nothing wrong with being 40 pounds overweight and that in any case, one glazed doughnut won't make any difference.

With self-hypnosis, what we are trying to do is *balance* all these negative factors coming from outside sources and irrational habits, with some positive thinking that comes from the real *you.* Some people, perhaps, do not need any help in this department. Their motivation and their determination is so great that once they make up their minds to stop eating irrationally, all those negatives seem to disappear. Unfortunately, I am not one of those people. Are you?

To enter into a state of altered awareness in order to accentuate the positive is more common than you may think. When you take a special person to a fine restaurant to enjoy a meal, you are entering an environment very carefully engineered to create an altered state of awareness. The dim lighting, the candles, soft music, the beautiful place settings and decorations almost instantly induce a feeling of well-being and expectation that is enjoyable in itself and also adds greatly to the enjoyment of the food.

When you turn off the lights and sit down to listen to your favorite music, you are soon in a kind of trance which vastly increases your appreciation of the music.

When you watch a football game in the midst of 50,000 cheering fans, your enjoyment of the play is likewise enormously heightened by the colorful, festive atmosphere.

Now picture yourself eating the very same food you got in that wonderful restaurant while sitting in your car, or listening to your favorite music while carrying a portable radio down the street, or watching that thrilling football game on a TV set in a bus terminal. . . . Not too much fun, is it?

Likewise, there can be a world of difference between reminding yourself to eat sensibly while you happen to be doing the laundry and telling yourself the same thing when you've induced a state of self-hypnosis. In the first instance, the suggestion, although perhaps made with utter sincerity, just doesn't have much effect. With self-hypnosis, what we're doing is creating the right mood for the advice really to mean something, to get down inside us where it will do some good, to make it *real.* And if you're willing to spend extra money to create the right mood for enjoying an evening out, why shouldn't you be willing to put a little effort (at no cost) into giving your reducing plan that same something extra?

But how, exactly, does hypnosis work? Many words have been written about this intriguing question, but the truth is that no one really knows. It seems, though, that hypnosis involves a kind of relaxation which enables us to become highly receptive to suggestions, so long as those suggestions are not disagreeable to us. You could say a lot more on the subject, but that's what it boils down to: a state of heightened receptivity to friendly suggestions.

There is no great theoretical gap between the kind of hypnosis which is induced by a trained hypnotherapist and the kind that you can induce by yourself. The professional, of course, is more likely to succeed, but not necessarily because his "powers" are any greater than yours. It's simply a matter of technique and experience, like so much else in life.

Of course, the professional hypnotherapist — who is probably a psychologist, physician, or dentist — frequently uses hypnosis to deal with problems which are more acute in nature than overweight. You may be interested to know, before trying your own brand of hypnosis, that these professionals have successfully used hypnosis to relieve intractable pain, greatly reduce the distress of childbirth, and quickly resolve problems such as bed-wetting and tobacco addiction. One of the most dramatic demonstrations of the power of suggestion is seen in the demonstrated ability of hypnosis to permit some hemophiliacs — bleeders — to undergo rather serious oral surgery without shedding a drop of blood. That may sound hard to believe but it's absolutely true. Clearly, if hypnosis can alter something as fundamental and physiological as blood clotting, its potential to alter mere habit is vast indeed. (Then again, some of us may feel that teaching our gums not to hemorrhage is child's play compared with teaching our teeth not to nibble, nibble, nibble!)

Formulating your goal. Let's get ready, then, for our first session of self-hypnosis. And interestingly enough, the very first and most important thing that needs to be done is the very same thing that we find ourselves doing over and over again as we follow the principles of sensible eating — thinking and planning.

If you induce self-hypnosis without already knowing what work you want to do during that session, you're probably going to mess up. It's the same as if you sat down to a desk full of papers without knowing what task you wanted to accomplish, or waltzed into your kitchen and began making dinner without having any idea what it was you really wanted to eat.

The goal you decide to work for during any given session of self-hypnosis should have three characteristics. If even one is missing, the session will not be worth much. Fortunately, formulating the right kind of goal is easy once you understand these characteristics.

First, your goal must be expressed in vivid, concrete imagery. In other words, you have to be able to see yourself doing something very clearly. You may, for instance, work on an image of yourself sitting at the luncheonette counter where you and your friends eat lunch every day, and you're saying to the waitress, "Ethel, I'll have my usual — a tuna salad and egg on toast — but please hold the potato chips." And as you picture this, you're also in touch with your feelings at the imagined moment, and it's quite clear that you're very comfortable about ordering that way, because you're asking for exactly what you want — no more, no less. You see yourself eating the sandwich, juicy, delicious, and satisfying. Every mouthful is enjoyable.

It won't do, though, to try to imagine something like "eating sensibly," or going through a holiday season without snacking, because these are very general, diffuse concepts, rather than specific images. Understanding the difference between the two takes us to the very heart of the process I call Super-Positive Thinking.

Images are what make self-hypnosis work. Even when you have entered the very relaxed and receptive state which makes self-hypnosis possible, words alone make very feeble tools. Somehow, our behavior is largely immune to the influence of mere verbiage. Advertisers know this, and that is why they're more than willing to spend huge sums of money to put their messages on television, even if they are able to reach audiences through radio at much less cost.

Exactly why this is so isn't easy to say. Which shouldn't be very surprising, since our understanding of how the human brain works and how it affects and is affected by behavior is — well, rudimentary would be a generous term. Recently, though, some very interesting experimental work has suggested that the answer may have something to do with the observation that the two sides of the human brain — left and right — have different jobs. These observations suggest that the left hemisphere of the brain is concerned largely with logic and rationality, among other things. Its language is words and numbers, and it comes into play most when we are balancing a checking account, reading a legal contract, or trying to figure out if we can get to see three more cities for less than $200 and if so, can we still be home by the evening of October 15. By contrast, the right side of the brain is believed to be largely concerned with the likes of images, color, melody, and rhythm.

No activity, of course, is exclusively concerned with the "left brain" or "right brain." In fact, if you're working on a project which mostly involves just one side of your brain, you can often get better results by inducing the rest of your brain to help out. Experiments with schoolchildren in eastern Europe have shown that retention of classroom material is much better when the work is summed up in the form of a melodic song. Better learning has also been observed in stroke patients who are learning to speak again when the words and phrases are reviewed melodically.

These examples may seem rather unusual, but good writers know that their message gets across much more forcefully and more lastingly when sensuous qualities are added to cold logic of everyday words. A poor writer would say "The farmer had gotten himself a haircut and he looked neat." William Faulkner says: "He has been to town this week: The back of his neck is trimmed close, with a white line between hair and sunburn like a joint of white bone." You *know* that the farmer has had a haircut — you can see it, practically feel it. A poor writer would say "The ocean glistened as the sun sank beneath the horizon." Robinson Jeffers says the same ocean looks "like a great stone someone has cut to a sharp edge and polished to shining." That's so good it's almost better than the real thing. And that's the kind of vivid immediacy you should strive for in formulating the messages you are going to give yourself under self-hypnosis.

The combination of advanced planning of each session and the "poetry" you use to bring your images to life make a powerful combination, uniting the left- and right-side functions of your brain in a way that will enable you not only to *think* positive, but to *feel* positive.

But a vivid image is not enough. The image-message you give yourself must also be *appropriate and realistic.* Again, this requires a little thought. Would it be realistic to see yourself sitting down to dinner, eating only a small salad, and feeling satisfied? Probably not — unless you happen to be in the habit of eating enormous lunches. Nor would it be realistic to see yourself jogging ten miles every day when in fact you haven't even developed the walking habit. On the other hand, it might be perfectly realistic and appropriate for you to see yourself walking to and from work if the distance is not greater than a couple of miles.

It's also a good idea to work only with images of new behavior that you know you'll be able to live with on a long-term basis. Don't waste time trying to rev up your mental engines to propel you on a 12-mile hike on Memorial Day. And needless to say, don't encourage yourself to skip meals that you're used to eating, or to do anything else that is grossly out of step with your life-style or instincts.

To achieve the third necessary quality, be sure that all your messages are *positive.* At one time, there was a lot of interest in conditioning people hypnotically to be revolted by whatever it was they were trying to avoid — cigarettes, pastry, or whatever. But there is now a kind of consensus among therapists that better long-term results are obtained when the suggestions are strongly and exclusively positive.

You remember that when I gave the brief example of ordering a sandwich without the ordinary potato chips, I didn't say that you should picture yourself thinking bad thoughts about those chips. Rather, I suggested you see yourself feeling very comfortable and satisfied with your favorite sandwich. We don't even want to say an unkind word about those potato chips: negative thoughts have a way of springing back at you like a rattlesnake chased into a corner.

Even when dealing with something as "real" as severe chronic pain, some therapists will *not* suggest that "you won't feel the pain anymore," or even that the pain will be less than it was before. Rather, they will probably work with images of profound muscular relaxation in the area involved, images of the involved tissues shrinking somewhat, becoming smooth, very smooth and pleasantly cool. They might suggest that the nerves in that area are very pleasantly asleep, or anesthetized. Note that all these variations are pictures of something being, or happening, rather than something not happening. Of course, some sensations of pain will be inevitable, but the therapist can teach the patient to interpret these messages in a different way. For instance, it might be suggested that occasionally, you will feel something unusual going on in your shoulder. It might be a kind of tingling, or heat, or a passing spasm. Suggestions would be given for dealing with these sensations.

The important thing going on here is that the word "pain" is never used, nor are there any images of pain being fought off. Super-Positive Thinking gives only tacit recognition to negative thinking; it does not stoop to quarreling with it.

I've used pain control as an example, because somehow it illustrates the principle of the positive approach very dramatically. But we're only concerned here with weight reduction and control, and for these purposes the moral in all this is that you should:

- *never tell yourself that you are not hungry;*
- *never tell yourself that you aren't going to eat this or that;*
- *never tell yourself that chocolate candy is full of mold.*

There are innumerable ways in which you can make your reducing program more successful by using positive suggestions. You can, for instance, see yourself filling up on delicious, vitamin-packed vegetables, see yourself going for a brisk 15-minute walk at breaktime, see yourself eating small portions of food at a restaurant so that you will feel thoroughly satisfied yet wonderfully comfortable and light at the conclusion of the meal, and so on. But more of that later. Right now we are going to learn how to put ourselves into the right frame of mind to mobilize all this creative positive energy.

Inducing self-hypnosis. The first time I tried self-hypnosis, I was doing just what you are: reading a book. It was actually the manuscript for a book, but no matter. As soon as I read the first brief description of how it can be done, I became so excited that I jumped up from the kitchen table, went into the bedroom, turned off the light, lay down, and 15 minutes later found myself delightfully hypnotized. The manuscript I was reading was entitled *Healing with Mind Power* and was subsequently published in 1978 by Rodale Press. Some time before, I had met the authors — physician Rich Shames and psychologist Chuck Sterin — in Mill Valley, California, and I'd been very impressed with the techniques they used to involve individuals with their own healing and well-being. I especially liked the fact that both of them used hypnosis as only one tool in a total or holistic approach to personal health improvement. I asked them if they would write a book on the subject for Rodale Press, and the manuscript I was reading at my kitchen table was the result. In fact, most of what I know about self-hypnosis I learned from Shames and Sterin.

At the time I read their manuscript, I was already about a month or two into my reducing program, so it seemed natural to use self-hypnosis to further this program. The results were very gratifying. The techniques I'm going to describe now are those which I used, and which I subsequently taught to participants in our reducing workshops.

Find a quiet place away from any distractions. It might be a den, your bedroom, or your basement. Your chair should be comfortable and the lighting conditions dim or dark. Make sure you won't be disturbed by the telephone or sounds from the TV. You might want to kick off your shoes and loosen your clothing. If you are an early riser, you might even want to do it first thing in the morning, while you are still in bed and everything is still quiet. You can even do it before retiring, if you aren't so tired that you might fall asleep — and if you can find an unoccupied bed.

> *Take a couple of deep breaths. With each exhalation, feel how any residual tension is leaving your body. Let your belly expand with each inhalation and exhale slowly. It's amazing how much good three deep breaths can do you, isn't it?*

Those few breaths you took were priming the pump that is going to finish the job of emptying your body of muscular tension. You are breathing quite normally now, but with every exhalation still more tension is leaving your body with the air you expel. You can feel the large muscles of your legs growing limp and pleasantly warm. The muscle tightness that you need in your hips and back to remain erect is not needed now, and it simply flows out of your body. You can feel all your bones actually settling deeper into your chair or bed as your thighs and buttocks and back muscles give up this unneeded tension.

You aren't concentrating on breathing because it is not necessary. Your chest and your lungs are thoroughly relaxed and your breathing rhythm is precisely in tune with your new relaxed state. Now the day's tensions are being drained from your arms, your shoulders. And as the last vestiges of tension drain from your scalp and your face, your eyes close quite naturally. Your neck muscles give up the tension they no longer need, and as that happens your head feels quite heavy as it sinks and relaxes against your easy chair or pillow.

You're feeling beautifully relaxed now and it's a very enjoyable feeling. But even more pleasant is the knowledge that in a few more minutes you'll be five to ten times as relaxed as you are now.

Your right arm is at your side, relaxed. You are now going to do something with your arm that you will find very enjoyable: permit it to levitate.

Except that you are not going to make it rise in the way you normally would. Rather, you are going to program it, give it proper instructions, so that it will rise entirely of its own accord. When it does so, that will be a signal to you that you have achieved a new dimension in the control of your behavior and body, that you have achieved an absolute fusion of mind and matter, that you are, in fact, in a deep state of self-hypnosis.

Imagine now that the lower half of your arm is being pumped full of helium, a gas which is lighter than air. As the helium is being pumped in, the blood is leaving. The whole process of transfusion takes only a minute, and even before the minute is up you can feel that your arm is becoming lighter. It is totally relaxed, yet it seems to be pressing much more lightly against your chair or bed. . . . Now all the blood, every last drop in your lower arm, has been replaced with helium, the gas which is used to inflate giant blimps. There is so much helium in your arm that your skin is actually slightly swollen with its pressure. And this helium, in accordance with the rules of nature, is slowly but inevitably going to cause your arm to rise.

So far, we're maybe three or four minutes into our session, and unless you are unusually receptive, your arm is not doing anything very interesting yet. And it probably won't do anything too exciting for five or ten minutes. If nothing much seems to be happening after five or six minutes, don't give up — everything is probably proceeding just according to schedule. The first time I tried this, I was just beginning to get bored with the whole thing after six or eight minutes when first my fingers, then my hand, and then my whole arm from the elbow down began quite mysteriously to crank themselves upward. There seems to be a kind of delayed reaction here, as the brain's messages gradually infiltrate and take control of the target area.

Your arm is now thoroughly filled with helium — there is no blood, no bone, no muscle, nothing except lighter-than-air helium straining to get skyward.

It may need some help though, so after a minute or two, you notice that a huge helium-filled balloon some nine or ten stories high is floating into view. Around your wrist there is a strap and now a grappling hook from the balloon catches that strap and begins to tug your arm upward. Then all the ballast in the balloon is thrown overboard, unleashing the full and irresistible power of the helium, and you feel an astonishing tug at your wrist as the giant balloon begins to bob up and down, seeking to haul everything within its grasp to the high heavens.

You are still thoroughly relaxed, enjoying the show. It is quite impressive, as the balloon continues to tug at the strap around your wrist. Your arm may be taking its time about getting up, but inevitably it will, because it's only natural.

Now another balloon comes along, lowers its hook, and joins the act. Every half-minute or so, another balloon comes along until there is a whole cluster of them bouncing lightly against each other as they strain and tug, lifting your arm up with them. Now you can feel your arm beginning to rise. The sensation is quite delightful. It continues to rise as still more giant balloons attach themselves to the others, until there is a vast panoply of balloons above you, exerting enough power to haul a small house skyward.

Now your right hand is anywhere from six inches to a foot or more off your chair or bed. Once you are satisfied that your arm has indeed levitated, cut the balloons free, one at a time, and allow your arm slowly and naturally to return to its original position. You are now in a new and very interesting state of consciousness.

In reality, it may not make that much difference whether your arm has risen an inch or as far up as it can go. Even if your arm has scarcely budged, you still may have achieved the necessary state of relaxation and receptivity for autosuggestion. If this particular induction does not seem to work for you, there are many others, some of which we will mention later.

At this point, you are ready to begin the "work" part of your session. It will probably be much shorter than the induction phase. What I am going to describe below is what I actually visualized during my first self-hypnosis session. You can choose whatever message you want to give yourself, but you might get some tips about how to frame your suggestions from my own experience.

Now, see yourself sitting down to dinner. Some of your favorite foods are on the plate, which is filled but not heaped. See yourself eating the meal slowly, relishing the aroma, the taste, the texture of the food as you chew and swallow each mouthful. As you slowly work through the meal, your sense of satisfaction gradually increases until you have finished. At that point, your belly feels perhaps half-full, which is perfectly normal and desirable because it takes 20 or 25 minutes after you have stopped eating before your food gives you the sensation of fullness. Knowing, then, that you have eaten what you require, and what will make you feel best, you leave the table and go into another room to pursue one of your favorite activities. Whatever it is you choose — working in the shop, listening to music, or whatever — see yourself doing it very vividly and imagine that the feeling of fullness continues to increase in your belly until after 20 minutes you feel much more satisfied than you did before. There is enough food inside you to take you through the night easily and into the next morning.

After running that scenario through your mind's eye once, you might give yourself a brief narrative, something like this, as the film plays itself again:

> *"I am going to want to eat meals of moderate size. Because that is exactly what I desire, and what my body really wants. So when I eat them, they are going to be extremely satisfying to me. After I eat what I want, my stomach is going to feel very warm and happy and contented. Right now, I can visualize myself feeling exactly that way. My mouth will be very relaxed and serene. And that's the way I will feel throughout the evening. My body and appetite will be perfectly contented, because they are getting precisely what they need and want for perfect energy and well-being."*

Invent your own words to go along with your own scenario, and then play the whole thing over maybe two or three times. Each time you play it over, add a little bit more convincing detail, just as a director would do in perfecting a scene for a real movie.

Having done this, you are ready to conclude your sessions. This will take only about one minute.

> *Take several deep breaths. With each inhalation, a sense of increased alertness to your immediate surroundings grows upon you. After a few breaths, you are aware that you are in your lounge or your bed and that you are very comfortable. Very soon now, you will be coming out of your hypnotic state, and when you do, you will be fully alert and feeling wonderful.*
>
> *Begin slowly counting backwards from ten. Take a breath with each number and be aware that as you do so, you are becoming increasingly alert. As you reach the number seven, your eyelids are becoming lighter and want to open. As you reach five and then four, you become increasingly aware of your hands and your legs touching your chair or your bed and it will be good to be fully awake again. Your eyelids now have an irresistible urge to open and just as you reach one, they do open and you are fully alert, feeling refreshed and serene. For another minute or so you'll remain where you are until you're naturally ready to resume your normal activities.*

After I used that particular approach several times, during the course of about a week, I decided on another message that was probably even more effective — for the simple reason that I had had much more time to think about it. And you will notice, too, that it is much more specific than the first message. The more specific, the better.

> *Sometimes I feel that my mouth is itchy or dissatisfied, that it desires something. Since I've eaten within the last few hours, I realize that what I really crave is a glass of cool, clean water. Water cleans the palate, refreshes the throat, and feels good to the stomach. Ordinarily I don't drink enough water so it's no wonder that I desire more. So when I get one of these uneasy feelings, I'm going to get my favorite glass, which is sitting on the counter top, fill it up with good, clear water, and drink it. I can see myself doing that now, and when I have drained the glass I find that that simple glass of water was wonderfully satisfying and that everything from my lips to my stomach has been refreshed, cooled, and put to rest.*

With that particular message, I didn't bother to visualize myself drinking water from the cooler at work, because I had no problem there. My only problem was at home, where I would shovel food into my mouth to satisfy what was in real fact a craving for nothing but water.

Please don't think that you can fool yourself, though, into drinking water when you're really hungry. It won't work because it's not realistic.

During the next few days, you're going to spend a few spare moments here and there devising appropriate messages for your inner self. Here are just a few of the possibilities:

If your problem is late-night eating, after ten o'clock, you might want to imagine yourself becoming quite sleepy at that hour and going to bed. In the morning, you wake up early, bathe, and go for a very enjoyable walk while everything is still quiet. *See* yourself doing this routine very vividly, as a daily habit. (If you find it difficult to go to bed when you change your routine, you can use hypnosis simply to relax. After induction, use one of the "deepening" techniques we'll describe shortly, and give yourself a posthypnotic suggestion that on coming out of your session, you will soon sink into a deep and very restful sleep.)

Perhaps you walk by a bakery every day as you leave work and can't resist stopping in two or three times a week to load up on cakes. The wrong thing to do would be to imagine yourself walking past the bakery and not wanting to buy something. The more realistic and appropriate thing would be to visualize yourself taking a slightly different route home, because the one you have been accustomed to is harmful to your well-being. See yourself walking this new route, feeling much more secure, knowing that each time you go that route you are in fact becoming a healthier and more attractive person. (You might think that walking home a different way is so simple as not to require any help from self-hypnosis. But that kind of habit is exactly the kind of thing that most people find so difficult to change.)

Perhaps your problem is that you live in a house littered with snack foods which your children insist that you bring home. Before you even begin thinking about hypnosis, you should have already done several other things, such as restricting the times at which these snacks may be eaten, keeping them out of sight when they aren't being eaten, and selecting for purchase only those items which appeal to your children but not to you. Having done all that, you can then work on seeing yourself drinking water or tea, eating fresh fruit, or going for a walk when temptation might strike. Conceivably, you might even want to visualize yourself buying only one or two snack items at the store, explaining to your children that too much snacking leads to health problems and an unpleasant appearance, and then remaining quite calm as they proceed to throw a Class A tantrum.

As a general rule, you should only work on one situation per session. If there are several things you want to work on, give each message a good week to do its work before moving on to the next one. During that week, you might want to do two or three sessions. It isn't necessary to do self-hypnosis every night, and it might get boring.

It's also a good idea to use hypnosis to reinforce those behavioral changes which you are currently working on. If you are thinking about jogging only as a distant possibility, perhaps something that you might start after you can walk for a few miles without feeling bushed, don't use hypnosis to sell yourself on jogging. On the other hand, if you are able to jog, but are having a difficult time sticking to your program — which is very common during the first few weeks — it is perfectly appropriate to visualize yourself putting on your jogging outfit, going to a pleasant place, and enjoying the unique sensation of rhythmic, moderate exercise. It isn't necessary or even advisable to try to imagine yourself running much greater distances than you are at present. (If anything, you should do the opposite, because the most common problem with jogging — aside from losing interest in it before you reach that point where it becomes highly pleasurable — is overdoing things, either in distance or speed.) The important thing is to lay down the pattern of getting out to your jogging place at least three times a week. Once you're there, the rest is easy. But what you might want to do is spend just a minute or so visualizing yourself jogging, feeling very relaxed and very natural, and becoming more healthy, more energized, and more slender with every stride. Because that is exactly what will happen. But the important thing, to repeat, is to get into the habit of jogging or doing whatever other exercise you have chosen. The combination of properly planning your day, making your jogging clothes readily available, finding a place where you're comfortable, and then strengthening this new pattern with hypnosis is very effective.

More about induction and deepening techniques. The induction technique I gave initially may be rather overdrawn for some people, who will be able to slip into trance without going through all the imagery I described. If that's your case, fine. Eventually, you will probably find that as you do more and more inductions, you will be able to enter a trance state much more quickly and easily. You can help this process along by giving yourself the suggestion while in the trance state that the next time you induce hypnosis, things will go much faster.

Here is an alternative induction technique for those who do not care for the arm levitation induction, or who seem to be having problems with it.

> *Sit in a chair, a straight chair, with your back fully supported and feeling very, very comfortable. Hold your right arm (if that is your dominant one) straight out in front of you, parallel to the floor. Now feel your arm strangely growing heavier. Heavier and heavier and heavier. It feels as though your arm weighs 50 pounds and it is just getting heavier and heavier and heavier. Heavier . . . and heavier . . . and heavier. Now your arm is quite naturally beginning to move toward your lap and the sensation is quite pleasant. As your arm continues to fall, you are aware that your eyelids are becoming very heavy also. Heavier and heavier. They are enormously heavy and they are growing heavier . . . and heavier . . . and heavier. Now feel your eyelids beginning to flutter as they begin to close. Soon your arm will reach your lap, and when it does so, you'll discover that your eyelids are also very pleasantly closed.*

You can see that that last induction is working with gravity instead of against it, which makes it a good technique for those who are somewhat resistant to normal hypnotic induction. The arm levitation technique is probably more effective in producing deep trance. However, the initial relaxation produced by the arm-lowering technique can be greatly amplified by using one of many deepening techniques.

> *Now that your eyes are closed, you are feeling wonderfully relaxed. What you are going to do now is to count backward from ten to zero, and when you reach zero, you will be much, much more relaxed than you are now. Ten . . . nine . . . deeper and deeper . . . eight . . . seven . . . much more deeply relaxed now . . . etc.*
>
> *Having reached zero, you are now in a very, very deep state of relaxation. But you are going to become even more relaxed, much more relaxed than you have ever been before. What I want you to do is search your memory for a time and place when you were beautifully relaxed (you should make this scene selection before beginning induction). Perhaps it was a quiet afternoon at the beach. If so, I want you to see yourself there right now. You* are *there, and you can feel the warm sun very deliciously toasting your body as a cool breeze blows in from the surf.*
>
> *It's the most supremely relaxing moment you've ever enjoyed. The warm sun, the fresh, clean air . . . it's wonderful and you're there right now. You give yourself up completely to the beauty of this moment . . . and as you do so, you realize that you are now in a very deep hypnotic trance. . . . You are now ready to begin the work of this session.*

As I describe these inductions and deepening techniques, I'm doing so as if I were instructing you. But of course, when you do them yourself, you'll be using the first-person voice. "I feel deliciously warm . . . just incredibly relaxed . . . I've never felt such a beautiful, peaceful moment." And seeing yourself very vividly in the scene you're creating.

Now, you may be asking yourself "How do I know I'm really hypnotized?" And the answer — from a very practical point of view — is that it doesn't really matter all that much. So long as you are deeply relaxed and giving yourself properly framed suggestions, you can be sure that you're not wasting your time. Look at it this way: innumerable scientific studies have shown that if you give a large group of people little white pills and tell them it's a new medicine that may help their digestion, their arthritis, or whatever is bothering them, approximately one-third of the people will experience symptomatic relief for varying lengths of time. Scientists call this the "placebo effect" and in some experiments, the rate of "placebo response" has gone higher than 50 percent. In fact, this phenomenon is so powerful that testing the true efficacy of new medications can be a very tricky business. In many experiments, the results achieved by using expensive and potentially dangerous drugs are only a few percentage points ahead of the placebo response.

Now, when people are given placebos, they aren't being hypnotized or even put into a state of relaxation. The process is helped, no doubt, by the potent ritual of a doctor handing out pills, and also by the patient's hope for relief. Yet, the whole transaction takes place in what is at least nominally a normal state of consciousness.

That being the case, you can see that the mind is so ready to accept "friendly suggestions" that the exact depth of your hypnotic trance is probably not going to be a crucial factor. Much more important, you should *believe* yourself when you tell yourself that you are in fact in a trance. Some people may run into problems here, because the first time they induce hypnosis, they simply aren't going to believe that anything unusual has happened. But as we said at the beginning of this chapter, being in a trance is not all that different from being in a normal state of deep relaxation. Your head won't be buzzing, and you won't feel that you're drifting through space. So just take your own word for it that you are hypnotized, and let it go at that.

To conclude this chapter, I'm going to take you through another self-hypnosis session, using a somewhat novel induction technique which I have used myself and found extremely effective. For the work part of the session, we're going to take a typical problematic situation and see what we can do about it.

To begin this session, sit comfortably in a chair, with your back comfortably supported and your eyes lightly closed.

> *In my mind's eye I see someone who looks very much like me sitting in a chair exactly like the one I am sitting in. His eyes are open and his arm is out straight in front of him. He appears to be extremely drowsy and it's hard for him to keep his eyes open. He's very, very drowsy and has an irresistible urge to sleep. His eyelids are beginning to flutter now, and his arm is wavering. His eyelids feel very heavy, very heavy and he just can't keep them open any longer. Now they're beginning to close. And his arm is*

falling, too, irresistibly falling. He is so drowsy, so tired. He must feel that his arm is enormously heavy. . . . Now, finally his eyelids are closed . . . and as he gives in to his drowsiness, he very pleasantly allows his arm to fall slowly downward until it is hanging limp at his side.

Now he's just sitting there, settling into his new state of wonderful relaxation. I'll just sit here, too, and enjoy the same delicious relaxation. . . .

Now he is going to make his arm levitate and I can sense that his arm is incredibly light, as if it were filled with helium. I can see his arm beginning to rise now . . . it is so light . . . it just wants to float. And now I can feel my own arm rising just as I see his arm rising and it's a wonderful feeling to let myself go. His arm keeps rising, I can see it, and I can sense that it's getting lighter and lighter, rising higher and higher. Up and up . . . higher and higher . . . lighter and lighter . . . lighter and lighter . . . just floating so pleasantly and effortlessly higher and higher.

Now I can tell that his hand will soon be reaching up toward his chin, and as it does, it will naturally fall very gently against his chest. I can see his hand getting closer and closer now and finally it is straight up and now it's beginning to fall slowly towards his chest. And when it just lightly touches his chest, he is going to be in a very, very deep state of self-hypnosis. . . . And how interesting that I can feel my own hand doing the same thing, and now it is falling very slowly and naturally toward my chest and now it just grazes my skin and as it touches me I am in a very deep state of self-hypnosis.

Now I will let my hand just freely and naturally fall into my lap, and when it touches my leg, I will be even more deeply in trance. . . . Now my hand touches my leg and I am much more deeply relaxed than I have ever been before.

Now I am especially sensitive to positive suggestion, and I am going to do the work that I came here for.

When I come home from work there is a lot of pent-up tension bouncing around inside of me. That's only natural. So what I'm going to do is use that tension to do something really enjoyable, that will work out the tension and really set me up to feel good the rest of the day. I can see myself now coming home and when I enter the house, I go straight to the bedroom and change my shoes. Then I'm going to get myself a nice, cool glass of water, which will be very pleasant. I can see myself doing that and I know it feels good. Now I can see myself leashing the dog. Both of us really want some exercise and we're both going to enjoy it.

I'm on the street now, heading for Ninth Street, and from there I go up to Elm Street and into the park. I see myself walking through the park and it's really good to be outdoors after a whole day at work. The dog and I are both very glad to be out there stretching our legs and getting some fresh air. And the more I walk, the more I enjoy it. The more I walk, the more relaxed I become. It's really great to be outside after a day at the office.

We're walking home now, and we both feel loose and comfortable after half an hour outside. I deserve that exercise after a day's work and I need it, too. It helps me feel better, think better, and work better. I can see myself doing that every day, and I notice that I'm slimmer than I used to be. Yes, definitely more slender. In fact, I've had to get a new pair of pants. I look younger, and there's a very youthful spring in my step. I like the way I look and the way I feel. That's the real me. An active person, who really enjoys walking. . . . That's something to look forward to every day, getting outside and walking. There I am, going down Elm Street, right at home, feeling good, and looking slender. Just the way I naturally ought to look. And I like looking that way.

Now, I'm going to return to being fully alert. As I'm sitting here, I can feel myself growing more in touch with my surroundings and I have an urge to open my eyes. My eyelids are becoming very light. I'm going to count down from ten, and when I reach one, I'm going to be fully alert. Ten . . . nine . . . my eyelids feel very light . . . eight . . . seven . . . more and more alert . . . six . . . five . . . my eyelids are feeling very light now and springy and they're going to open when they reach one . . . four . . . three . . . feeling very alert now and ready to go . . . two . . . my eyelids are open now . . . one . . . wide awake and fully alert.

The idea in that particular session was not only to get primed for a walk that is going to use up about 200 calories, but to break a habit pattern of mindless eating which habitually occurs when you come home from work. But please note that nothing in this session can be construed as an attempt to kid yourself. It *is* perfectly normal to be tense upon coming home from work. The logical way to get rid of that tension *is* to go for a walk. Walking outside *is* enjoyable and you *do* enjoy it more after you've been walking for about 15 minutes or so. Another bonus is that upon returning from your walk in a more relaxed state, you'll be in a much better state of mind to eat rationally.

That was just one example of autosuggestion. Design your own suggestions to deal with your specific needs, using your own images and your own words. But here are some general principles to keep in mind:

- *know beforehand what message you are going to give yourself;*
- *know also what induction technique you're going to use and what kind of deepening technique, if any;*
- *frame your suggestion in vivid, concrete terms . . . see and feel yourself doing what you want to do;*
- *make your suggestion realistic and appropriate;*
- *express your suggestion exclusively in positive terms;*
- *work on one suggestion per session;*
- *use your suggestions to help carry out your consciously made plans, and plan consciously to carry out your suggestions.*

Appendices

A

Questions and Answers

Our diet workshop participants had many questions both before and after reading portions of this text. In this section, I'll try to answer some of the most commonly asked questions, admitting that a number of them — even some important ones — are only touched on lightly or ignored altogether in the main text.

Q. Aren't people with chronic weight problems "different" from other people, physically and psychologically? Your plan doesn't seem to give much recognition to these differences I've read about.

A. The answer to your question is yes, no, and maybe. That seems to be the "consensus" of current medical research, at any rate. In fact, when I began writing this book, I had intended to write a whole chapter on this subject, but as more and more research came out, it became obvious that the research results were so conflicting that to emphasize these supposed differences which exist in overweight people would only cause confusion.

If you put together all the differences some researchers see in chronically overweight people, you would come up with a scenario something like this:

As a baby, the obese person was probably introduced to solid foods at too early an age and overfed as well. It's likely he or she had overweight parents, who not only pushed their eating habits on the baby, but perhaps passed along some genetic tendency to obesity as well. The result was that the baby not only became too heavy, but actually created millions of new fat cells to accommodate that extra weight.

When the chubby baby became older, he or she could not play as vigorously as other children. Probably the extra weight discouraged activity, while the lack of activity encouraged still more weight gain. Still later, during the teenage years, the future-fatty probably ate too much again, and created still more new fat cells. And that is very important (or so the theory goes) because those extra fat cells will be hauled around for the rest of the person's life. That will make it easier for fat to be stored and may even create a kind of "hunger for fat" that the person with fewer fat cells does not experience.

Continuing with this amalgamated and simplified version of supposed differences in obese people, the overweight person probably has hormonal imbalances as well. Many overweight people have abnormally high circulating levels of insulin, which stimulates the appetite and then encourages incoming nutrients to be stored away as fat rather than quickly burned. There may also be a tendency to have a lower basal metabolism rate, so that carrying out the everyday business of body chemistry, breathing and pumping blood, requires fewer calories than these jobs do in the normal person.

Psychologically, the overeater frequently turns to food to satisfy feelings of loneliness or depression, or simply as a means of coping with stress. He also responds to food in a more superficial way, and is likely to eat greatly excessive amounts of food when that food is served in a very attractive or enticing way. (In contrast, this theory holds, normal people simply eat until their hunger is satisfied and then stop.)

Finally, at least one well-known researcher has theorized that many overweight people subconsciously *desire* to be heavier than they should be. He observed that many people who lose a lot of weight and then gain it back, return to *exactly* the same weight they were before they began dieting. Why? He suggests that in some way this higher weight must seem "natural" to the person. If not his mind, then his body chemistry, perhaps, is happier being (for instance) exactly 47 pounds heavier than normal.

Most of these theories and observations are supported by scientific evidence. They also enjoy a certain popularity, perhaps because overweight people feel better "knowing" that their fatness really isn't their fault, and also, perhaps, because doctors and scientists enjoy the feeling that they understand the true nature of what is often called today's most common health problem.

Despite all of that, there is an *equally* convincing body of current research which demonstrates that these so-called "differences" are just a lot of nonsense, and as misleading as they are false.

It's possible, even likely, for instance, that the "new fat cell" theory is largely a result of mistakes in research techniques. While new fat cells may indeed be created, this contrary opinion holds, that creation may occur during any period of life, not just infancy or adolescence, and the importance of those new fat cells in creating obesity problems is probably insignificant anyway.

Likewise, there are good studies showing that obese people do *not* eat under stress any more than nonobese people, nor do they respond to food "cues" in a manner different from their slender friends. And if the fat person's metabolism tends to be sluggish, that's almost entirely a result of the fact that he gets very little exercise. A change in life-style would remedy that situation almost overnight.

Researchers who favor the notion that fat people are basically the same as everyone else tend to believe implicitly in the principles of this book. That is, they believe that fat people are fat simply because they eat too much, and they eat too much not because of any overwhelming physical or psychological mechanisms, but simply because they lack the skills and habits of sensible eating.

My own feeling at the moment — which is subject to change as yet more research results come in — is that while there *are* probably certain "differences" in chronically overweight people, they are not the major cause of obesity in about nine out of ten cases. I don't really think, though, that the true significance of these "differences" can be understood except in the context of holistic health, which emphasizes the interrelationships between such things as behavior, appetite, metabolism, diet, and so forth. And what I suggest is that most people can greatly modify these so-called differences or "givens" by modifying various aspects of behavior.

In other words, your circulating insulin levels *may* be somewhat high, but they can be reduced by eating more fibrous foods. They can also be reduced by exercise. Your metabolism *may* be sluggish, but you can speed it up with exercise. And maybe you *do* have a powerful tendency to react to food in an irrational way, but you can modify that, too, by consciously changing your behavior, which will immediately begin to weaken and eventually all but extinguish those irrational responses.

Q. If obesity is, as you say, the most common health problem in

industrialized countries, how can it be that medical science hasn't yet come up with the answer to these basic questions about the causes of obesity? Why is there so much conflicting evidence and confusion?

A. It *is* ironic that scientists seem to know more about bodies in the far reaches of space than they do about their own bodies. Perhaps that's just the problem — the closer you are to something, the more difficult it may be to understand it. At any rate, *all* nutritional research, not just obesity research, is fraught with confusion and controversy.

To appreciate why that is so, consider that the bulk of nutritional research is actually carried out on animals, usually rats, and the results obtained can never be directly translated to humans. But even when the research is carried out on human beings, the subjects studied are often from highly specific population groups, such as young, healthy college students, hospitalized patients, or very obese people, so the results obtained may be no more applicable to people in other population groups than the data obtained from rat studies.

Also, the methods used by various scientists doing similar studies are different, and there's always the likelihood that their different results are nothing more than a reflection of their different techniques. The results obtained from a weight-loss study lasting for one month, for instance, may be totally invalidated when another scientist carries out the same study for six months. What's more, most studies are carried out under highly artificial conditions, with food intake being strictly controlled. When a similar study is made using a population group living freely and normally, the results are often totally different.

Hopelessly complicating the entire picture is the fact that each individual is unique and is involved in a complex relationship with such unpredictable factors as psychological stress, major or minor illnesses, changes in life situation, and so forth.

Consequently, many people now believe — and I count myself among them — that many of the "hard answers" we once expected to get concerning human health may not only take a lot longer to discover than previously thought, but may *never* be pinned down in the same way as problems in the purely physical sciences. Hard and fast answers seem especially elusive when we attempt to use them to advise people how to behave to achieve a certain goal. Real life is not only a long way from laboratory science, but in another dimension, and that goes even for the real life of the scientist working in that laboratory.

That doesn't mean that we can't be helped in some way by scientific research. But it does suggest that we should regard the results of that research not as "facts" but as insights, clues, and helpful hints worth trying. Everyone involved in personal behavioral research is a perpetual pioneer.

Q. I went on a diet five years ago and after losing 15 pounds, it seemed like most of the weight came off my bust. My face was a little thinner too, but there was hardly any change at all in my arms and hips. What can I do to make sure that I lose weight in the right places?

A. Have you ever heard of "spot reducing?" I've seen many articles about it in women's magazines, and some reducing spas feature it in their advertisements. But as far as I've been able to determine, spot reducing is about as real as low-cal pie in the sky.

You'd *think,* wouldn't you, that if you exercise your arms a lot, or your hips or your thighs or your stomach muscles, that the fat in those areas would be preferentially broken down to provide fuel for adjacent muscles. Only it doesn't work that way. When your body is forced either through exercise or by a deficit of incoming calories to call for fuel from its fat banks, it chooses the branch where it's going to make its withdrawal according to a scheme known only to itself. If you do a lot of hiking, most of the work is being done by your leg and back muscles, but the fat you burn up may well have come largely from your chest or arms. Or, you could do a lot of rowing, lose ten pounds, and discover that you've lost two inches from your waist.

You also read a lot about "toning up" this area or that area of your body, suggesting that the fat in that area is somehow either going to disappear or shrink. But I can tell you from personal experience that doesn't happen, either. When I was 25 or 30 pounds heavier than I am now, I used to do a lot of exercise but paid no attention at all to how much I was eating. I used to do hundreds of sit-ups at a time, sometimes as many as a thousand. And my stomach muscles became hard as rocks — if you could find them under all the blubber surrounding my midsection, which you couldn't.

However, the fact that there is no such thing as spot reducing most definitely does *not* mean that you can't get your arms and hips to shed that excess fat. All you have to do is to *keep* reducing until you reach your ideal weight, which would be something approximating the values found on weight-height charts. When you have reached that weight, it's almost certain that your entire body will have been normalized. Have you ever seen a person who is genuinely slender — at their ideal weight — in every part of their body except one? I haven't — with the possible exception of some women who are genuinely slender except for an especially generous bosom. It is possible, of course, that you could be reasonably slender all over except in one place, where you are *slightly* larger than normal, because that particular area happens to be the last hold-out of your fat reserves. If that's the case, the next few pounds you lose will almost certainly be withdrawn from that area.

But without exception, all the people I have seen who tell me they just can't do anything to reduce in a certain spot are substantially overweight in *more* places than that one spot. In order to trim down that one spot, they first have to get rid of the excess fat they're carrying on the other parts of their body.

Q. Does that mean there is no point to doing calisthenics or other kinds of exercises, except to burn up calories?

A. No. Despite what I said before about doing sit-ups, I recommend them strongly (always to be done with knees fully bent) because what makes bellies hang out is not only the blubber around them, but poor tone of the underlying muscles which permits the abdominal contents to protrude. When you do a lot of sit-ups, or strengthen your abdominal muscles some other way, as by leg lifts or kicks, those muscles tighten up and hold in your gut. That will not only improve your appearance, but take a lot of strain off your lower back as well. When you see relatively skinny people who have pot bellies, what you're usually looking at is a little extra fat wrapped around very weak abdominal muscles.

Strengthening the other muscles of your body will also help improve your posture, and to the extent that your posture is good, you will look better, and somewhat more slender.

Q. In the community where I live, it seems that many of the women are quite a bit overweight. Most of these women have jobs, many of them in factories, and they do housework too. You'd think they'd be burning up a lot of calories and stay slender. Why is that, or is it just a coincidence?

A. It might not be a coincidence. Researchers at the University of Michigan, who studied almost five thousand adults in the city of Tecumseh, found that education and socioeconomic status seem to play a role in conditioning the eating habits of people. Specifically, they found that women who did not go through high school, or only attended for a few years, tended to be considerably fatter than women who had at least 12 years of schooling. But education itself seemed to be less important than economic status. There were indications that women who did not have much schooling but who married into higher-income families tended to be much leaner than similar women who married working-class husbands.

Curiously, the exact opposite trend was found in men, with relatively well-to-do men being fatter than working-class men. But the difference between women was greater, with the most educated women weighing about 11 pounds less than women with only a grade-school education. That difference is not a result of smaller height, either, because the wealthier women averaged only 26 percent body fat, as opposed to 32 percent for the less-educated women.

We can't say for sure why this trend occurs, or even if it holds true in other communities besides the one studied. It's my impression, though, that it is a general tendency, and I would guess that the reason for it is simply that wealthier women place more importance on being slender.

Ethnic factors may also play a role. Some communities simply seem to enjoy eating more than others, and probably more important, do not see anything wrong with being 20, 30, or 40 pounds overweight. On the contrary, they may believe that being well-padded is a desirable quality. A few generations ago, some historians point out, it was almost a status symbol to be fat. Slenderness was associated with not having enough money to eat well. Perhaps some people still feel that way.

None of this means that your education, wealth, or ethnic origins *determine* whether you will be fat or slender. It does mean that your family, your friends, and even your community can *influence* you in your eating habits. Call it peer pressure if you want to, or social feedback, or simply example. The milieu in which we live plays an important role in influencing how far we go with our education, what our aspirations are, how early we marry, how many children we have, and what our life-style will be. But many people who find themselves in a given milieu simply reject some of the values they see around them and substitute their own. To be realistic, people who do this usually have a high degree of motivation.

What I'd like to say to you, then, as a person living in that community, is that you should not be afraid to have values which are different from the people around you, and that you should make sure that your motivation is kept at a high level. It would be an excellent idea for you to seek out other people in your community who *share* your values — in this case, the desirability of being healthfully slender — and help keep each other motivated. In fact, that is a good principle regardless of what community you live in and regardless of what your unusual values may be. People who want to exercise should seek out people who already *are* exercising regularly. Probably the best way to do this is to join an appropriate club. It's not only a great way to motivate yourself, but to make new friends as well.

Q. If I overeat one night, at a party, for instance, what should I do? Skip a meal the next day?

A. It is perfectly normal, and absolutely acceptable, to overdo food once in a while. By once in a while, I mean no more than once a week. Giving yourself permission to do that means that you aren't chained to a certain eating program, and that you can always look forward to an occasional splurge. In the long run, it's really not going to affect your reducing or maintenance program very much at all. What's more, the less you worry about it, the more likely it is that your natural appetite control will work automatically the next day to reduce your intake of food.

Q. You didn't say very much in your book about overweight children. What can we do to make sure our children don't become fat, or to help them reduce?

A. The principles and techniques explained in this book will work equally well for children as for adults. Usually, getting children down to normal weight is *easier* than doing the job with an adult for the simple reason that most kids do not have the money to go into a store and come home with boxes of pastries, cases of beer, and gallons of ice cream. *If you have no junk food in your house, don't use sweets as a reward, and don't keep nagging your child to eat, there should be no great difficulty.* Every time I have seen a fat child, I have seen parents whose behavior needs modification, with the most common error being offering and reoffering the child food he doesn't need.

Many parents who claim that they have to buy junk food because the children "demand it" are deceiving no one but themselves: what they're really doing is using their child as an excuse to bring home junk food so *they* can eat it too!

Other parents seem intimidated by their children and let them buy or eat anything they want. I would strongly suggest that such parents seek help from a counselor or psychologist. Or better yet, a relative or parent whose children are slim. What that friend might tell them is that it's perfectly OK for kids to squawk, complain, nag, even cry, holler and tell you they hate you. Kids act like that for all sorts of reasons. And although I'm no psychologist, I do know that the major purpose behind 90 percent of that whining and nagging is the desire to have the parent establish firm limits on what the child can get away with. Children *need* limits, they *need* discipline. They crave it, it's an integral part of their development. But there's no kid on the face of the earth who *needs* potato chips and bottles of pop.

If you have trouble handling that approach, consider how your daughter is going to feel about you when she's 17 years old and weighs 150 pounds. And remembers how you gave in to her infantile whining for sweets — which her high school psychology course will probably have taught her was nothing more than a disguised request for discipline and love.

Sure, I know that kids will eat junk at their friends' houses and can buy their own candy bars. But I doubt if one child in a hundred is going to get fat that way.

More advice: don't try to ingratiate yourself with your child by bringing home gallons of ice cream or boxes of snacks. There are better ways to express love. Don't urge the overweight child to take seconds or keep asking him if he's had enough to eat, just because your parents always did that to you. Don't tell him he can have ice cream or a snack if he's a good boy or girl. And if he doesn't feel like eating at all, or only plays with his dinner, what's wrong with that? Why not let his natural appetite control express itself? And if you have to throw out his food, fine! (See "Trash Your Fat!")

Q. If I'm not mistaken, you didn't say to check with your doctor before going on a diet. Is there a reason, or did you just forget?

A. It would be easy for me to say, "Check with your doctor before beginning any diet," which is what everyone else seems to say, and then wash my hands of any misfortune that may befall you. But in all sincerity, if you are substantially overweight — 25 pounds or more — it is, at least in my opinion, much more important for you to go to your doctor and ask his permission to keep doing nothing. By doing nothing, you may well be increasing your chances of developing heart disease, high blood pressure, diabetes, arthritis, gout, low back problems, or problems with your feet. By following the reducing program outlined in this book, which involves losing no more than five or six pounds a month, and does not involve the elimination of any class of foods, not even junk food, it is extremely unlikely that you will be endangering your health.

On the other hand, if you are thinking of launching into one of the traditional diet plans, which usually involves eating between 800 and 1,200 calories a day, you *should* seek medical advice before doing so, as that caloric intake may represent a drastic and sudden change for you. Ironically, if you do go to a doctor to seek advice about dieting, it's likely that he will recommend that very sort of diet.

Having said that, I will back off a little and suggest that if you have a chronic metabolic disorder, such as diabetes or gout, you should not only check in with your doctor before beginning a reducing program, but keep in touch with him as things progress. You will be told, for instance, that if you have gout and go on a crash diet, you may suffer severe pain for the first few weeks as uric acid crystals are suddenly liberated. And if you have maturity-onset diabetes and are on insulin, your insulin requirements will probably be reduced as you lose weight. Many people with that form of diabetes find they can go off the hormone supplements completely when they have normalized their weight. But it is important to take neither too much nor too little insulin, so your condition should be monitored regularly.

Q. What about kneading your fat to loosen it, so that you lose it faster?

A. That seems to be a fairly well-established belief, although it's fading rapidly. And it should fade, because as far as I know, there's nothing to it. By shaking your fat, pounding it, rolling it, slapping it, or thumping it, about the only thing you will accomplish is to rupture some blood vessels. If you are extremely overweight, or prone to circulatory problems, you might even do worse.

The one thing you *can* do to encourage your body to burn fat is to exercise regularly. Active people burn fat much more readily than sedentary people.

Q. What can I do to avoid lots of loose, sagging skin after I lose weight?

A. To a very large extent, the body takes care of that naturally. However, when you lose 50 pounds or more, there is probably going to be some noticeable extra skin — although it probably won't show unless you are wearing a skimpy bathing suit. I must admit that I don't know of any exercises or special techniques to avoid that. In severe cases, plastic surgery is sometimes carried out.

Q. Which is more important to cut out of the diet, fat or sugar?

A. An ounce of sugar has about 110 calories; an ounce of fat, about 250. A tablespoon of sugar has about 45 calories; a tablespoon of cooking or salad oil, 120. On the average, between 40 and 50 percent of all the calories in a typical American diet come from fat. It's conservatively estimated (by defenders of sugar) that sucrose and other refined carbohydrates which are *added* to foods comprise another 25 percent of dietary calories.

Perhaps the best way to go about reducing the amount of fat in your diet (you don't want to eliminate it totally because some fat is vital to health) is to trim meat of visible fat and sharply reduce the use of fried foods, butter, mayonnaise, and salad dressings. The best way to cut back on sugar is to avoid cake, candy, and soda pop. If you cut back on the sugar in your coffee and still drink soda, you're kidding yourself, because a 12-ounce bottle of soda contains the equivalent of more than nine teaspoons of sugar.

Q. Many doctors say that even when you're dieting, you don't need vitamin supplements. They claim that unless your own doctor recommends them, vitamins are a waste of money. Could you explain again why you recommend supplements?

A. Deciding how you should spend your energy in the pursuit and protection of health and well-being is a very interesting process. And money is simply another form of energy, representing work you have already done, which has now been "translated" into an extraordinarily flexible, exchangeable form.

Your question has led me to calculate that during the last 15 years or so, I have spent approximately $3,500 on life insurance premiums. Having just checked my pulse, I suddenly realize that all that money has been totally wasted (plus another good chunk I could have earned in interest). . . . Or has it?

That is not really an impertinent question, because speaking "scientifically," it *has* been wasted. And what about my health insurance policy? My property insurance? My automobile liability insurance? My special travel coverage? What about my smoke detector? My burglar-resistant lock? I'd be hard-pressed to demonstrate that those cash outlays weren't "wasted," too.

So you see, most of us spend considerable portions of our precious energy in efforts to protect ourselves (and our families) against a whole array of potential dangers, and using nutritional supplements as a kind of health insurance is just one more way in which we do this. No doctor can justifiably make the statement in print or on TV that *you* do not need supplements, any more than a financial advisor writing in a newspaper can tell *you* how much insurance you need. If either of those experts were to meet you personally and spend considerable time examining your special needs, he could give you some potentially very useful advice, although he still couldn't give you *answers.* Quite possibly, *you* put a higher value on your own health or peace of mind than these experts do. And if you are highly concerned about your present and future health, you might want not only to take some supplements, but do regular exercise, avoid food additives, drink purified water, and so forth. None of these things has ever been "proved" to prevent illness or lengthen your life, but there's no incontestable proof that any other program of self-protection or self-improvement is guaranteed to pay off, either.

All of the above are a kind of philosophical answer to your question. The physical or biochemical part is, I hope, adequately dealt with in the main text. Keep in mind, though, that my attitude toward the need for nutritional insurance is influenced by the observation that the great majority of people who want to lose weight have a history of crash dieting. And because they are relatively sedentary, the total amount of food they can eat is quite limited. In the process of shortchanging themselves calorically, they can come very close to shortchanging themselves of vitamins and minerals as well.

Q. Isn't the high-protein diet the best way to lose weight? Many people say it is. I have a friend who has lost 40 pounds so far on the high-protein diet, and when I was on it myself, I lost 20 pounds in just a little bit more than two months — before I went off the diet and gained all the weight back.

A. No, I don't think the high-protein diet is the best way to reduce or to maintain your weight. And for several reasons, some of which have only been revealed by research within the last year or so.

First, although weight loss during the first few weeks on a high-protein diet is definitely more impressive than when eating a mixed diet, it's been discovered that almost all the difference is a result of water loss. But you can only lose so much water, so eventually that rapid weight loss slows down.

There are different ways of interpreting that. Some people think it's good, because the rapid weight loss during the first month can be very encouraging. In contrast, when eating a regular or mixed diet, no weight loss at all may be experienced for the first week, because the water is temporarily retained, and that can be discouraging. (It's also one reason why I advise strongly against weighing yourself every day.)

On the other hand, what happens when people on the high-protein diet discover after two months that the same diet which was initially causing them to lose four or five pounds a week is only producing a one- or two-pound weight loss now? Maybe they think they're not dieting carefully enough and cut back their calories still more, only to find that the difference hardly shows up on the scale. That, too, can be very discouraging.

One of the supposed benefits of the high-protein diet is that it produces a mild state of metabolic ketosis, and as a by-product of that process, certain chemical substances called ketone bodies are created which are said to suppress appetite. However, whether or not that really happens, or whether the effect is lasting, has now been seriously questioned.

Another theoretical benefit of the high-protein diet is that it "spares" body protein, some of which is always lost along with body fat when dieting. But that also has been called into question. The most recent study I've seen, in fact, reveals that eating a mixed diet actually spares *more* protein than a high-protein diet, although the difference is not statistically significant.

But the biggest objection I have to the high-protein diet is that it is *unnatural.* As you know by now, I don't believe in any diet plan which forces you to eat in a radically different manner than you're accustomed to. Eventually, either when you give up, or reach your desired weight, you are going to go off the high-protein diet and revert to the same old eating patterns that made you overweight to begin with. And there is evidence that when you go off the high-protein diet, you may put your excess weight back very rapidly indeed.

Q. Does it make any difference what *time* of day I eat?

A. If research carried out a few years ago at the Chronobiology Laboratories at the University of Minnesota can be confirmed by other studies, it could make a very significant difference indeed. What that research indicates, in a nutshell, is that food may be less fattening when eaten earlier in the day than when eaten in the evening.

The three university scientists (all of them named Halberg) have established quite a reputation for their research into the importance of innate body rhythms and the physiological effects of doing various activities at different times of the day. One research finding of interest to them was that when mice, normally active during hours of darkness, are permitted to eat only at the beginning of their usual activity span, they tend to weigh less than when permitted to eat only in hours of early light, a time when they are normally inactive.

Are these results applicable in some way to human beings? To find out, the Halbergs put a group of seven human beings through pretty much the same routine. In one experiment, they prepared meals that contained 2,000 calories and served them to the subjects either as breakfast or dinner. In either case, that was all they were permitted to eat the entire day. At the end of the week, the subjects who had eaten the meal for breakfast had all lost weight, while those who ate the very same meal for dinner showed either a smaller loss or a gain in weight. The breakfast-only group lost an average of 2.5 pounds more than the dinner-only group.

That experiment was somewhat artificial in design, not only because the calories were limited, but because the food was selected by the scientists, and some of it was not to the liking of the participants. But a second experiment was a little more lifelike. This time, the subjects were told that they could eat whatever they wanted and as much as they wanted — the only rule was that they had to eat everything either for breakfast or for dinner. Six weeks later, after all the subjects had gone through both early and late routines, it was revealed that eating everything for breakfast rather than dinner resulted in a greater weight loss of 1.4 pounds per week.

Now, losing more than a pound a week while eating whatever you want, and as much of it as you want — even if all of it has to be crammed down in one meal — may strike you as being a very exciting possibility. It even sounds a little bit like the basis of the next fad diet. But before you get too excited, keep in mind that it would be very difficult indeed for the average person to eat just one meal a day. And before putting too much confidence in these findings, I would want to see them duplicated by scientists at several other research centers, for experience has taught me that conflicting results are more the rule than the exception.

Nevertheless, I think there's an important lesson here. And it's most applicable to dieters who practically starve themselves all day, only to give in finally late at night and demolish hundreds of calories in a matter of minutes. Not only are these people needlessly torturing themselves, they may actually be doing themselves a caloric injustice by doing their eating so late, when food might be, in effect, more fattening.

On the positive side, it might be a good idea to try to *gradually* shift more and more of your eating to the earlier hours of the day. Try it, at least; give it a chance, and see what happens. But don't try to do it all at once, because eating an enormous meal for breakfast when you aren't used to it can ruin your whole day. Neither am I suggesting that you make a meal of six eggs and four pieces of toast. Eat some vegetables, soup, stews, even meat. Perhaps after a month or so, you will find that breakfast is your largest meal of the day, lunch a little smaller, while dinner is something light, like melon and cottage cheese, or even a couple of eggs and toast.

There may be a bonus in that kind of regimen, because it's been postulated by a heart specialist that eating late at night may predispose certain people to a dangerous blood clot while they are sleeping, when the fatty contents of a large dinner are absorbed into their sluggish blood stream. It's better, according to this theory, to eat your biggest meal earlier in the day, so that when the food is absorbed, some seven hours later, your blood circulation is relatively active, and better able to cope with the sudden influx of fat.

But maybe when all is said and done, the most attractive thing about eating a greater percentage of our food earlier in the day is that, as daylight-active creatures, it's probably more *natural* for us, just as it's natural for nocturnal creatures such as mice and owls to eat during darkness.

Q. Is it natural to gain weight as you grow older?

A. No, it's natural to *lose* weight as you grow older. That's because our muscle mass diminishes as we grow older, so if we stay at the same weight, a higher proportion is actually fat. That will be even more true if you have not done any vigorous exercise in your mature years to try to hold on to your muscles. I know people in their sixties who weigh the same as they did in their twenties, when they were trim and muscular, but who are very obviously fat and flabby today.

Q. But don't people usually gain weight as they grow older? And is that because their metabolism is slowing down, or because they are less active?

A. In America and other developed countries, there is a tendency for people to put on weight as they put on years. But that trend does not seem to hold in other countries, such as India and China. When I recently traveled through the Caucasus region of the Soviet Union, I noticed that the people there who live to enjoy a very long and healthful life remain slender regardless of their age.

It's true that metabolism does tend to slow down a bit with the advancing years — about 2 percent every ten years — but the effect of that is insignificant compared to the lessening *activity.* The trouble is, many people do not reduce their food intake as their caloric expenditures go down. It's much better for older people to do everything possible to remain active, rather than to keep cutting back on their calories, because eventually it will be difficult for them to satisfy their protein, vitamin, and mineral requirements. In advanced age, it may no longer be possible or advisable to climb a lot of stairs, carry heavy packages, and do other chores which burn up calories rapidly. But that doesn't mean it's necessary to be sedentary. Walking slowly and comfortably on a level sidewalk or path will burn up those calories just the same. It may take longer, but it will be a lot safer.

Q. My husband isn't making things easy for me. He keeps asking me, "When are you going to stop this stupid diet?" How should I handle that?

A. A good reply might be: "This is my new way of eating."

The worst possible reply would be something like "*You're* the stupid one! Don't you want me to lose weight?" That's bad for two reasons. First, you're insulting your husband, and that's the wrong thing to do for someone on a diet, because experience shows that support from a spouse can be one of the most important factors in determining whether or not you are successful in losing weight.

The second thing wrong with that reply is the question "Don't you want me to lose weight?" Both you and your husband should understand right from the beginning that you're losing weight because *you* want to lose weight. Too often a spouse will reply that he or she does *not* want you to lose weight. A common remark is "I love you just the way you are!" There is a subtle implication there that he or she may not love you or will love you less if you *do* lose weight. What the real motive behind that kind of remark is, I can't exactly say, but I do know that in a great majority of cases, the initial reaction of scorn and mockery soon changes to one of new respect and admiration. And not infrequently, after you have lost a substantial amount of weight, your spouse suddenly become interested in slimming down, too.

But it's vital for both of you to understand that your losing weight has nothing to do with his feelings. You're doing it strictly for *your* sake, because *you* want to, because you're convinced that's what you want. But don't be too rough in getting this point across.

I like the statement, "This is my new way of eating," because it's very neutral. It doesn't make any statements about his faults, your desire to please him, or anything really controversial. Further, it emphasizes the fact that you aren't on a temporary diet, but that you have adopted new habits of eating which are more closely in tune with your natural appetite and your best health interests.

Q. I've used some of the positive thinking techniques you've suggested, but after three months, it's becoming harder for me to stay motivated. Do you have any tips?

A. One technique that helps many people is the self-reward system. Make a deal with yourself that if you lose a certain amount of weight by a certain date, you'll reward yourself with something really meaningful. Your goal should be reasonable, neither too demanding nor too easy. A loss of six to eight pounds over a period of two months might be appropriate. If you reach that goal, be sure not to renege on the bargain. Go ahead and be good to yourself. Do something out of the ordinary. Buy some exciting new hobby equipment, a health club membership, or camping equipment. One of the best gifts is new clothing, because it's probably going to be in a new and smaller size — a perfect recognition of your accomplishment as well as a reward for your efforts. Believe me, there is nothing more pampering to the ego and strengthening to your resolve than to be able to fit into a size that you haven't worn in years. In fact, you may be *forced* to be a little indulgent with yourself, because as you progress, your old clothing simply won't fit you. After you lose 20 or 25 pounds, you may well find that even your shoes are too big on you.

In my own case, my trouser size went from a 36 to a 31, my shoe size from a 9 to 8½, my sport shirt size from a medium to a small, and my dress shirt from a 16 to a 15½, which has to be cut full-trim to fit me. That can be an expensive proposition, but the boost to your motivation when you see how good all that new clothing looks on you is well worth it.

It's also helpful to realize that in the course of losing weight, it's perfectly natural for you to hit a plateau every now and then. There were many weeks when I thought I was following my program fairly well, but my weekly weigh-in showed no progress. I told myself that the important thing was to follow the program, not to play games with the scale. And I usually found that the next week, or sometimes the week after that, I would suddenly lose four or five pounds, even though I hadn't done anything different. The name of that game is water retention, not willpower, so don't let it discourage you. That's why I advise against getting weighed more than once a week, and against setting short-term weight-loss goals.

Another good way to keep up your motivation is to get more exercise. This afternoon I took a long, slow walk through the park to admire the fall foliage, and then through the prettiest section of town to admire the homes and landscaping. I didn't work up a drop of sweat, but that walk made me feel *good* — fit, relaxed, and pleased with myself. The fact that it burned up hundreds of calories and actually reduced my appetite for dinner wasn't as important as the psychological effect. Taking long walks is a very obvious physical way of reminding yourself that you are a new person, a very fit and active new person.

Q. I've lost 22 pounds and I'm very happy about it, but lately I notice that I've been waking up earlier than usual, about a quarter after six or six-thirty instead of seven. That doesn't really bother me, but I wonder about it. Is it good, bad, or just a coincidence?

A. More than likely, it's simply because when you lose weight, you require less sleep. That has been shown in scientific studies, and was also true in my case. Why heavier people require more sleep is not understood, but we can speculate that the less body mass that has to be restored and refreshed, the less time is required to do the job.

Q. Someone told me that you can drink all the alcohol you want and never get fat because your body can't turn alcohol into fat. That sounds ridiculous, but he insisted that he was right.

A. He *was* right . . . but only partly, and the part that doesn't matter. Yes, it's true that the body cannot convert the calories in alcohol into fat. All it can do is "burn" those calories for metabolic energy. But your friend is dead wrong in asserting that you can drink all you want without getting fat. Here's why:

When your body begins burning alcohol as fuel, it *stops* burning its normal fuel. The result is that ingested food calories which would ordinarily be burned to keep you breathing and moving are stored away as fat. A few drinks before dinner and a few after are more than enough to insure that your entire dinner will be banked as blubber.

Q. Is it possible that doing exercise can make you *gain* weight? I read that muscle weighs more than fat.

A. It's true that a handful of muscle weighs more than the same handful of fat, but there's no way you're going to add that much muscle to your body in the course of losing a handful of fat. Young men can add muscle mass quite readily; older men more slowly. Young women, no matter how much they exercise, even if they lift weights, cannot bulk up their bodies with muscle as much as their male counterparts can; it's a matter of hormones. And older women will add even less muscle mass. Strength, most definitely, but not bulk.

Q. I have gone on a diet several times, and it wasn't all that difficult for me to stick to it, even though I was only eating 1,200 calories a day. But what I *couldn't* do was keep the weight off, after I'd lost it. Why was that? Shouldn't it be the other way around?

A. During the *reducing* phase of your diet, you were eating less than you were permitted to eat during the maintenance phase which followed. But even though you were eating less, your motivation was probably at a very high level and you were extremely conscious of what you were eating. You had a kind of temporary obsession, really. When we are in that kind of state, we can draw on enormous reserves of energy. There is also a strong sense of purpose to what we are doing, and we feel ready to sacrifice almost anything in order to reach our goal.

But what happens once that goal has been reached, when you have lost your 20 or 30 or 50 pounds at the end of your diet? Suddenly, there no longer seems to be a sense of purpose to your eating behavior other than enjoyment. While losing weight seems to be something positive, maintaining your weight is somehow negative and rather dull. So our sense of purpose and motivation can disappear almost overnight.

Another factor is the tendency toward a big let-down after any concentrated period of effort: physical, mental, or emotional. Whether you have been dieting, studying for finals, or redecorating your house, once the big burst is over, the big poop-out begins.

Add to all of the above the fact that when you are on a strict diet, you're also building up feelings of deprivation, and you can see why the "success" you had in crash-dieting (that's what a 1,200-calorie diet is, really) could not be maintained over the long haul.

I think we can all see from the above why it is wrong — so *absolutely wrong* — to set out on a weight-reduction plan with the idea in mind that your problem is that you're X pounds too heavy, and that success will have been reached when you lose X pounds. That kind of thinking practically insures that you'll regain much of what you lost. If, on the other hand, you have a very clear idea that your goal is to *change your behavior,* and in so doing, lose weight naturally, there is no big poop-out.

Q. Does losing weight affect your sex life?

A. It certainly *can*, either positively or negatively.

If crash-dieting leaves you feeling tired and irritable, it's obviously going to have an undesirable effect on your sex life. And not just for physical reasons, but because your irritability may alienate your spouse and strain *all* aspects of your relationship. Losing weight sensibly, however, can only help your love life. You are bound to have more energy. You will even require less sleep. You will also look better — and feel better about how you look.

Recently, there have been indications that dieting can in some cases increase a man's level of testosterone — the male hormone. Men who are quite obese often have elevated levels of the female hormone estrone, which is created from a precursor in fatty tissue. Estrone is believed to suppress production of testosterone in the testicles. In one recent experiment, dieting reduced the level of estrone in 15 obese men to normal, and caused an increase of testosterone to the normal level in all except 2. The men in this experiment lost an average of 45 pounds, and were on a diet severely restricted to only 320 calories a day, so it isn't possible to say to what extent these findings would be applicable to all overweight men who reduce.

B

Calories Burned by Various Activities

If you enjoy paying compulsive attention to numbers, you are better off lavishing your energy on the calories burned by exercise than on the calories contained in food. You can only manipulate your diet so much, cut back so many calories, before you begin to feel deprived and genuinely hungry. But if you manipulate your daily schedule to permit an extra hour of easy walking, you can burn, for instance, another 300 calories a day without having to worry about physical or psychological backlash. Sure, the first few days your legs will be a little sore, but after a week or so, there will be no strain if you are in normal health.

The table in this appendix is also useful in assessing, in approximate terms, the caloric costs of your daily routine. It's especially useful, I think, in pinpointing the effect of changing habits. Let's assume, for instance, that you are a 48-year-old woman and that you are now considerably heavier than you were 25 years ago, even though you're convinced you're eating less than you used to. But perhaps as the years passed, you changed your routine in a number of seemingly minor ways. Looking at the table, you'll be able to see what effect these changes have had. Back then, you might have gone dancing once a week, which would have burned up about 220 calories. You went bowling once a week, which burned up another 150 calories. On weekends, you waitressed for a total of 12 hours, which consumed 2,280 calories. The kids were home then, so you did a lot more housework, and in those days, you used to hang your wash out on the line, which burns more calories than using a drier. You estimate the weekly decrease in "housework calories" at 400. Add it all up and your total decrement on a weekly basis — compared to what you expended at age 23 — amounts to about 3,050 calories.

Of course, you aren't spending all that additional time sleeping, but instead of hanging out wash, scrubbing floors, and bowling, your new activities are more in the line of driving a car, sewing, and watching TV. If you add up the additional hours which you now spend in such activities, you might come up with a total of, say, 850. Subtracting that from 3,050 gives you a net weekly exercise decrement equivalent to 2,200 calories, or about 315 a day.

And what do those 315 extra calories a day mean? Quite precisely, they mean about 22 extra pounds of weight. Remember that every extra pound of fat you're carrying causes you to burn up another 14 calories. So to find out at what point your added weight will cause you to stop gaining weight, you would only have to divide 315 by 14, which turns out to be 22.5.

So much for diagnosis. Now let's talk about *cure.*

Bowling no longer interests you, you say, and you'd need a team of draft horses to pull your husband out to a dance. Neither does scrubbing floors nor hanging out your wash especially appeal to you. Well, what about swimming? If you swam at the rate of only 20 yards per minute, which is an extremely slow pace, permitting frequent rests, you could burn up — assuming that you now weigh about 150 pounds — some 150 calories in half an hour. Do that three times a week and you're subtracting a total of 450 calories. What about walking? Three miles an hour is a very comfortable pace, and if you walk for an hour four times a week, that's another 1,200 calories. And let's say that you return to the piano you've forgotten about, and substitute an hour of piano playing every day for an hour of TV watching. That's another 280 calories a week. All of which gives you an additional 1,930 calories a week, enough to produce a weight loss of 19 pounds. If, at the same time, you reduce your daily food intake to the tune of 300 calories a day, the losing won't stop until you have lost 40 pounds, which will take you very nicely back to where you were 25 years ago. But long before you reach that level, you will have gained so much new energy that you'll be walking more, swimming more, and probably enjoying many other activities as well, which will speed your weight loss along that much faster.

A word or two about the technical side of this table is now in order. First, the caloric values given *include* the calories you are burning up as a result of your Basal Metabolic Rate, frequently referred to as the BMR. Those are the calories that you spend on such basic chores as circulating your blood, breathing, and digesting your food. The average figure usually given for the BMR is about 50 calories an hour — essentially the same number of calories expended when sleeping, when you aren't doing anything but your BMR act. If you are considerably overweight, your BMR will naturally be higher, but 50 is a useful approximation.

That means that when the table says that if you weigh 150 pounds and walk for an hour at 3 mph, you'll burn up 300 calories, what it really *means* is that you'll burn up 250 calories *more* than you would by doing nothing, which burns up 50. That difference would possibly appear to be serious if you use these figures to calculate the additional calories (above normal calorie expenditure) you'll be burning through exercise. In other words, an hour of walking is only burning up an *additional* 250 calories, calories that you wouldn't expend if you were watching TV, not 300. However, these higher values are so commonly used that I have used them myself throughout the book. There is, though, a saving grace that in many cases will make up the difference — and maybe even more — very nicely.

Edward Watt, Ph.D., cardiovascular physiologist at the Preventive Cardiology Clinic in Atlanta, Georgia, told us that in calculating the calories burned by exercise, it's important to add the time to return to the preexercise resting rate. *Because the increase in metabolic rate can continue for from 30 minutes to several hours after exercise is discontinued, the number of calories consumed by the exercise is significantly greater than this table indicates.*

That was quite a revelation to me, actually, and it explains why vigorous exercise seems to produce weight loss beyond what you'd expect, while very light exercise, like ironing, which does not really raise your metabolic rate, seems disproportionately small in its effect. Moral: to the extent that your exercise gets you sweating, it's giving you a calorie-loss bonus, by burning fuel even after you've showered.

Be aware also that the values given here are, quite naturally, approximate, and they depend largely on the degree of vigor with which the given activity is pursued. Also, if you do not pursue a given activity for one solid hour, simply divide by two for half an hour, three for 20 minutes and so forth.

Calorie Costs per Hour of Some Common Daily Activities

	Weight (in pounds)		
Activity	110–125	150	180–200
ASSEMBLY LINE WORK			
Light	150–175	220	260
Medium	205	260	305
Heavy	230	295	340
BRICKLAYING	160	205	235
CALISTHENICS	235	300	350
CARPENTRY			
Light	150–180	175–230	200–270
Heavy	280	355	415
CHOPPING WOOD			
By hand	355	400–450	525
Power saw	175	220	260
Stacking wood	300	380	400–440
DANCING			
In general	240–250	270	300–450
Light	215	275	320
Rock	195	250	295
Square	330	350–420	480

Equivalent Activities and Remarks

1 hour of light carpentry or making beds.

1 hour of scrubbing floors or waitressing.

¾ hour bicycling at 10 mph, hiking at 2 mph with 20-lb. pack, or tennis (doubles); 60 minutes of walking at 3 mph.

½ hour of chopping wood by hand or 1 hour of cutting wood by power saw; 1 hour house painting; 2 hours of typing.

1 hour hiking with 20-lb. pack at 2 mph; ½ hour of handball; 1 hour swimming at easy pace. For optimum fitness, calisthenics should be combined to use muscles of the whole body in order to be as valuable as swimming, tennis, handball, etc. Begin with relaxation and limbering routine to warm up; after workout, use relaxation techniques again. Main disadvantage is that calisthenics can be boring unless done in groups or to music.

1 hour washing and polishing car; 1 hour driving a truck; 20 minutes of handball; 35 minutes of walking at 4 mph.

1 hour of volleyball; walking 4 miles in an hour.

2 hours of cutting wood with power saw.

½ hour of chopping wood by hand; 25 minutes of handball.

1 hour of gardening; 1 hour of golf, carrying clubs.

1 hour of gardening; ¾ of an hour bicycling at 10 mph. Calorie expenditure for dancing usually falls in the range of 270–460 and is governed by tempo of the music as well as individual style and enthusiam.

Calorie Costs per Hour of Some Common Daily Activities

Activity	Weight (in pounds) 110-125	150	180-200
DOMESTIC WORK			
Baking	107	137	162
Cleaning windows	180-195	210-250	295
Dinner preparation	105	135	155
Ironing	160	205	235-240
Making beds	165-200	210-240	245-300
Scrubbing floors	195	250	295
Sewing, knitting	75	95	110
Shopping	130-150	165	195-200
Washing and drying clothes			
Washing machine	125-150	160	190
Using dryer	125-150	160	190
Hanging on line	190	245	285-300
Washing dishes			
By hand	105	135	155
Dishwasher	60-85	110	130
DRESSING, UNDRESSING, WASHING, SHOWERING, BRUSHING HAIR	150-160	205	235
DRIVING A CAR			
Light traffic	60-75	95-100	110-115
Heavy traffic	80-105	100-135	155-180
DRIVING A TRUCK (tractor-trailer)	180	230	270

Equivalent Activities and Remarks

35 minutes of easy cycling; 15 minutes of rope skipping. Values are less if using a mixer, more if beating batter by hand. Many recipes require both.

1 hour hanging clothes on line; 25 minutes of rope skipping; 3 hours of TV watching.

Basically the same as for standing only, unless you are whipping eggs, flipping a pizza shell, bending and opening drawers, etc.

2½ hours of TV watching; 50 minutes of waitressing. Ironing burns up considerably more calories than just standing, due to lifting and pushing the weight of the iron and hanging pressed clothes.

1 hour 10 minutes of walking at 2 mph; 1 hour of yoga; 1 hour washing and polishing car; ¾ hour swimming or calisthenics.

Floor scrubbing *can* burn up to 420 calories per hour.

About the same as reading. Both slightly more than just sitting watching TV.

This is light shopping. Carrying heavy packages will increase calorie loss by 100.

Modern equipment makes household tasks easier today, but it may not seem that way if you are not physically fit.

In most cases, one hour per day is taken up by these activities.

Higher values are for standard versus automatic transmissions.

1 hour washing and polishing car; 1 hour raking; 20 minutes light snow shoveling; 50 minutes easy rowing.

Calorie Costs per Hour of Some Common Daily Activities

	Weight (in pounds)		
Activity	110–125	150	180–200
GARDENING			
Weeding, hoeing, digging, spading	240–305	300–390	400–450
Raking	175	220	260
HOUSE PAINTING	165	210	245
LAWN MOWING			
Push power mower	210	270	310
Sitting mower	115	145	170
PIANO PLAYING	95	120	145
READING	70	90	105
ROPE SKIPPING (75 skips/minute)	435	555	645
RUNNING			
5½ mph (easy jogging)	515	655	760
8 mph	625	800	930
11 mph	955	1,220	1,420
12½ mph (very fast)	1,220	1,550	1,805
SEX			
Foreplay	80	100	115
Intercourse			
Vigorous	235	300	350
Easy	105	135	155

Equivalent Activities and Remarks

Attitude and zeal will dictate variations in calories lost here. 220 to 300 calories/hour is a good rule of thumb, if you are hoeing beans or pampering azaleas.

¾ hour tennis (doubles) or hiking at 2 mph with 20 lb. pack; 22 minutes of handball or light snow shoveling.

1 hour cleaning windows, light assembly line work, or light carpentry; ¾ hour tennis (doubles); 2¾ hours TV watching.

Pushing your mower instead of sitting on it will burn up almost *twice* as many calories.

A lively piece such as Liszt's "Tarantella" requires ⅓ more energy than Beethoven's "Appassionata" and 2½ times as much as Mendelssohn's songs.

Burns same amount of calories as writing, slightly more than just sitting or TV watching, and less than typing.

1½ hours of walking at 4 mph or volleyball; 7 hours of TV watching. Do this as a "coffee break" to get your energy up and to avoid the doughnuts and Danish. Running shoes are advisable to avoid ankle and knee damage.

How far you run is more important than how fast you run. Unfit people should design a stretching and calisthenics program for themselves before taking up running in order to avoid knee pain, back pain, or muscle strains.

Burns slightly fewer calories than typing.

Same as hiking or swimming for the vigorous approach or piano playing for the easy approach.

Calorie Costs per Hour of Some Common Daily Activities

Activity	Weight (in pounds) 110-125	150	180-200
SITTING	60	80	90
SLEEPING	50	65-80	80
SNOW SHOVELING (light)	475	610	710
SPORTS			
Bicycling (geared bike, average terrain)			
Easy pace—5 mph	190	245	280
Moderate pace—10-12 mph	240-325	270-415	300-475
Vigorous—13-15 mph	515	660-720	760
Bowling	150	190	240
Fishing			
From boat	105	135	155
Wading	235	300	350
Golf			
Twosome, Carry clubs	295	380	440
Twosome, Pull clubs	260	335	385
Foursome, Carry clubs	210	270	310
Foursome, Pull clubs	195	250	295
Handball	470	600	695

Equivalent Activities and Remarks

1 hour TV watching; 6 minutes of handball; 20 minutes of light assembly line work or carpentry; 15 minutes of gardening; 13 minutes of walking at 4 mph.

Also equivalent to lying awake in bed. Does not vary much from Basal Metabolism Rate.

1 hour handball; 2 hours walking at 3 mph; tennis (doubles); or swimming at 20 mph at 20 yds/minute.

Energy cost of sports are approximate, influenced by the vigor of the individual participant.

If you cycle six miles to and from work instead of driving, taking about 30 minutes each way, you could burn 15 to 20 pounds of fat in a year.

This is regular bowling rather than continuous bowling. Possibility of taking in more calories in food and beverages than are burned up makes bowling a doubtful weight-loss activity.

40 minutes of slow walking; 25 minutes of swimming or calisthenics.

½ hour of hill climbing; 1 hour of calisthenics.

Not much better than walking unless you carry your clubs, play on a hilly course, or jog around the course before each round. If you use a caddie or electric cart, forget it!

2 hours of walking at 3 mph; 55 minutes of vigorous rowing or moderate swimming; 8 hours of watching TV. A vigorous workout provides a maximum of exercise in a minimum of time. Remember to warm up first.

Calorie Costs per Hour of Some Common Daily Activities

Activity	Weight (in pounds) 110–125	150	180–200
Hiking, 2 mph (20 lb. pack)	235	300	350
Hillclimbing	470	600	695
Horseback riding			
Walk	130	165	195
Trot	325	415	475
Rowing			
Easy	235	300	350
Vigorous	515	655	760
Skiing			
Downhill, excluding lifts	465	595	690
Cross-country (5 mph)	550	700	800
Swimming			
20 yds/minute	235	300	350
35 yds/minute	425	540	630
55 yds/minute	660	835	975
Table Tennis	355	360–450	525
Tennis (recreational)			
Singles	335	425	495
Doubles	235	300	350

Equivalent Activities and Remarks

4 hours TV watching; 3/4 of an hour gardening; 1 1/4 hours washing and polishing car; 1 hour of walking at 3 mph; 22 minutes of running at 8 mph; 1/2 hour of handball; 40 minutes of table tennis.

1 hour of handball; 55 minutes of moderate swimming; 3 hours of bowling; 1 hour of downhill skiing, excluding lifts; 1 3/4 hours of brisk walking.

1 hour of light shopping; 50 minutes of bowling or slow walking.

1 hour square dancing; 1/2 hour of running at 8 mph.

Easy rowing is equal to 1 hour of hiking at 2 mph with a 20 lb. pack or swimming at 20 yds/minute. Vigorous rowing is equal to 1 hour 8 minutes of handball or 1 hour of running at 5 1/2 mph or 1 hour of swimming at 45 yds/min. You will burn more calories in choppy water on a windy day.

Calorie cost is maximized by low temperatures. Excellent activity for fitness and endurance because skiing uses all major muscle groups. The amount of uphill skiing required by cross-country terrain will influence the number of calories burned.

Also uses practically all the muscle groups of the body. Should be balanced by some weight-bearing exercise such as running for all-around muscular development. If you cannot gauge your swimming speed, you can count on burning from 200 to 700 calories per hour. The butterfly stroke burns up the most calories; the crawl the least.

3/4 hour of handball; 6 hours TV watching; 1 1/2 hours of hiking at 2 mph with 20 lb. pack; 33 minutes of running at 8 mph.

Singles: 1 hour and 25 minutes of swimming at 20 yds/minute; 33 minutes of running at 8 mph.

Doubles: 1 hour of swimming at 20 yds/minute; 22 minutes of running at 8 mph.

Depends on how you play the game: if you run for every ball, you will burn more calories than an opponent who considers it a waste of time to run for a shot that will put him out of position.

Calorie Costs per Hour of Some Common Daily Activities

	Weight (in pounds)		
Activity	110-125	150	180-200
Volleyball (recreational)	275	350	405
Wrestling	620	790	920
STANDING	105	135-140	155
TV WATCHING	60	80	90
TYPING	80-90	105-115	120-135
WAITRESSING	190	245	285
WALKING			
2 mph	145	185	215
3 mph	235	300	350
4 mph	270	345	405
WASHING AND POLISHING CAR	180	230	270
WRITING	70	90	105
YOGA	180	230	270

Table prepared by Sharon Faelten.

Sources:

Astrand, Per-Olof, and Rodahl, Kaare. *Textbook of Work Physiology.* New York: McGraw-Hill, 1977.

Burton, Benjamin T. *Human Nutrition.* 3d ed. New York: McGraw-Hill, 1976.

Conrad, C. Carson. *How Different Sports Rate in Promoting Physical Fitness.* Washington, D.C.: President's Council on Physical Fitness and Sports, 1978.

Equivalent Activities and Remarks

1 hour of walking at 4 mph; 40 minutes of rope skipping; 1 hour 10 minutes of calisthenics; ¾ hour of chopping wood by hand.

Slightly less than vigorous swimming.

40 minutes of piano playing. The only activity which uses fewer calories is lying in bed and staring at the ceiling.

35 minutes of walking at 2 mph.

1 hour of washing and polishing car.

Calories burned by walking depend on type of surface (asphalt, grass, level, incline), type of clothing and wind resistance, as well as body weight. At approximately 3 mph, you burn 15% more calories walking on grass than on asphalt. Walking up a 15% grade burns up twice as many calories as walking on the level. Walking downstairs uses only one-third the calories of walking upstairs. *Running* upstairs demands even more calories. Climbing upstairs with a load, such as a basket of laundry, burns 11 times as many calories as walking on the level carrying the same load.

¾ hour of walking at 3 mph; 15 minutes of running at 8 mph; 25 minutes of rope skipping; 1 hour of raking; 25 minutes of handball.

Same as reading; slightly more than sitting or watching TV; less than typing.

Value is due to benefits of flexibility and relaxation. Recommended as part of a warm-up routine for more vigorous activities such as running or bicycling.

Guthrie, Helen Andrews. *Introductory Nutrition.* 3d ed. St. Louis: C.V. Mosby, 1975.

Kuntzleman, Charles T. *Activetics.* New York: Peter H. Wyden, 1975.

Kuntzleman, Charles T. *The Exerciser's Handbook.* New York: David McKay, 1978.

Oakley, Nigel. "Weight Control and Metabolism," *Cycling: The Healthy Alternative.* London: British Cycling Bureau, 1978.

Shephard, Roy J. *Frontiers of Fitness.* Springfield: Charles C Thomas, 1971.

C

Ideal Weight Table

The weights given here are those which have been associated with the lowest mortality, or to put it bluntly, the smallest chance of dying, and are therefore believed to be the most healthful weights. *Note that the heights assume that a man is wearing one-inch heels and a woman two-inch heels.* If you know what your height is in bare feet, add the appropriate number of inches to find your height in the table. If you usually weigh yourself without clothing, subtract several pounds from the values given, which assume that you are wearing clothes. The various "frame" sizes given refer to bone structure, not overall body mass. Look at, or better yet, measure the circumference of your wrists. Consider how wide your hip bones and shoulders are. Then compare these values to those of other people to get some idea of what your frame size is. If you are especially well-muscled, you can also consider that to be part of your frame. Generally, people over 50, unless quite muscular, should weigh in the lighter areas of the ranges shown.

Ideal Weights for Adults
(age 25 and over)

Height (in shoes)*	Weight in Pounds (in indoor clothing) Small Frame	Medium Frame	Large Frame
MEN			
5′ 2″	112-120	118-129	126-141
3″	115-123	121-133	129-144
4″	118-126	124-136	132-148
5″	121-129	127-139	135-152
6″	124-133	130-143	138-156
7″	128-137	134-147	142-161
8″	132-141	138-152	147-166
9″	136-145	142-156	151-170
10″	140-150	146-160	155-174
11″	144-154	150-165	159-179
6′ 0″	148-158	154-170	164-184
1″	152-162	158-175	168-189
2″	156-167	162-180	173-194
3″	160-171	167-185	178-199
4″	164-175	172-190	182-204
WOMEN			
4′ 10″	92- 98	96-107	104-119
11″	94-101	98-110	106-122
5′ 0″	96-104	101-113	109-125
1″	99-107	104-116	112-128
2″	102-110	107-119	115-131
3″	105-113	110-122	118-134
4″	108-116	113-126	121-138
5″	111-119	116-130	125-142
6″	114-123	120-135	129-146
7″	118-127	124-139	133-150

Height (in shoes)*	Small Frame	Weight in Pounds (in indoor clothing) Medium Frame	Large Frame
5′ 8″	122–131	128–143	137–154
9″	126–135	132–147	141–158
10″	130–140	136–151	145–163
11″	134–144	140–155	149–168
6′ 0″	138–148	144–159	153–173

*1-inch heels for men and 2-inch heels for women.

Source: *Statistical Bulletin,* vol. 58, October, 1977, p. 5 (New York: Metropolitan Life Insurance Company). Based on Build and Blood Pressure Study, 1959, Society of Actuaries.

D

Food Rating and Evaluation Guide

The main body of this book has been devoted to teaching you to become more conscious of when and why you are eating. The table in this appendix is devoted to raising your consciousness of *what* you are eating.

By now, you already know that it is very unrealistic to choose your diet solely on the basis of its calorie content. On the other hand, it can be *helpful* to know more about the calorie content and nutritional value of various foods and dishes. Using this knowledge as an information resource, rather than a strict guideline, you'll be able to make better informed decisions when it comes to choosing among foods you actually like.

There are a number of unusual features in this table along with the more familiar information, so some brief explanations are in order.

The arithmetic data is taken almost entirely from various publications of the United States Department of Agriculture, while in a few cases, values have been obtained from some other sources, such as labels. However, don't be too impressed with the precise accuracy of these figures, even though most of them are "official." What most people don't realize is that for the most part, the values given in government food tables are "representative," not absolute. The vitamin content of an apple, for instance, will vary somewhat depending on the variety, the weather during the growing season, where the apple was grown, when it was picked, and how long it was in shipment and storage before consumption. Government researchers evaluate data from numerous tests and come up with one convenient value. When foods are cooked, even more variables are operating, including the method of cooking, the maximum temperature reached, the length of cooking, and how quickly the food was consumed after preparation was completed. Small differences, then, between different foods in this table should not be given much importance, because in reality they are likely to be factitious.

Government researchers, I might also add, use teaspoons which are slightly smaller than most other teaspoons, with the result that the caloric value of a teaspoon of sugar, for example, is given here as 15, while in other tables you may have seen, the figure is 16 or even 18. Such differences are not really important and I only mention them in the event that you begin comparing data and discover that the values for identical amounts of the same food seem to vary slightly from table to table. You may also be slightly confused if you attempt to find some of the data presented here in government tables, because in certain instances I have done my own calculations to present values for more realistic serving sizes.

N/C rating. This is the abbreviation for what I call the Nutrient Value-Caloric Density Ratio. I developed this ratio as a means of expressing the fact that it isn't simply the number of calories that you should worry about, but what you are *getting* for those calories in the way of real nourishment. A bowl of chili con carne, by way of illustration, has a lot more calories than an apple, but you will notice that while I give an apple an N/C rating of only "Fair," chili con carne is rated as "Excellent." That's because the greater number of calories in the chili con carne more than pay their way by providing tremendously greater nutritional value.

Likewise, the banana is rated as "Good" while a cup of lima beans (usually considered a no-no to dieters) is rated "Excellent." While the cup of lima beans has almost twice the calories of the banana, it also has ten times as much protein, eight times as much calcium and five times more iron. The lima beans are also going to be more filling than the banana, which is another factor I tried to take into account in coming up with these ratings.

Keep in mind that these ratings are focused on the needs of the dieter, which may be somewhat different from someone else's needs. The apple we talked about before contains a goodly amount of pectin, which is helpful for someone trying to lower his cholesterol, but the pectin value is not considered in determining the N/C rating. However, the bulk and crunchiness of the apple *were* considered because, while not exactly giving greater nourishment to the apple, they nevertheless make it more desirable to the person who wants to give his mouth and stomach that satisfied feeling.

It hardly needs to be said that N/C ratings can be somewhat debatable. Although I tried to be as objective as possible, I'm certain that many of these ratings could still be justifiably criticized. In certain cases, I may have gone a bit overboard in one direction or another when the food involved enjoys a popular reputation which I don't think is particularly deserved. I doubt that many dieticians would rate apple juice "Poor," as I have done, but so many people abuse this beverage that I think anyone who regularly stocks it in the refrigerator needs to be shaken into realizing that it is far from being a health food.

Protein. Protein is to your body what wood is to a cottage, what concrete is to a skyscraper, and steel to a bridge. It is the most fundamental building material and plays a critical role in the structure of every tissue and organ of the human anatomy. Even your bones, composed mostly of minerals, require substantial amounts of protein to get all those minerals to hang together.

It is sometimes said that getting enough protein is no problem for Americans, but like so many other things said about the diet of the "average American," that statement can be dangerously misleading. And if you are a relatively small person watching your weight, you would do well to watch your protein intake also. In order to get enough protein to maintain your body in good repair (various parts are always being discarded and replaced) it is advisable for a woman to get between 40 and 60 grams and a man between 50 and 70.

The question is, what do you have to eat to get this amount? It might be instructive to glance at our table for a moment, and add up all the protein provided by typical servings of the first 15 items. Doing so, we discover that the total amount of protein contained in a large handful of almonds, a cup of chopped amaranth leaves, an ounce of amaranth grains, one apple, one glass of apple juice, one serving of applesauce, three raw apricots, a serving of dried apricots, a glass of apricot nectar, a serving of asparagus, half an avocado, two slices of bacon, one banana, one cup of green beans, and a whole cup of cooked lima beans amounts to a grand total of only 37 grams of protein — not enough for most people's daily requirement.

True, those items aren't exactly a typical daily diet, but there are people who, in an attempt to lose weight fast, eat almost nothing but fruits, vegetables, and grains. That in itself is not bad, providing these vegetable-source foods contain enough protein — protein which is properly balanced. In practice, that means if you are getting your protein from vegetable sources, you should always eat some grain products at the same meal you consume legumes such as beans, peas, limas, or garbanzos. Or consume nuts along with grain products. Otherwise, you will not get an efficient mixture of amino acids, the components of protein.

Just scanning the table, you will quickly see that a single serving of many meats or fish will give you more protein than all those other foods we mentioned put together. Eggs, cheese, and other dairy products are also rich in protein. Since virtually all lean meats, poultry, and fish are given very high ratings in the table, it does make a certain amount of sense to try to include one serving of them in your daily diet — unless, of course, you are a vegetarian. While in some instances a vegetarian will have to consume more calories to get high-quality protein than the person eating lean meat or fish, the vegetarian has the advantage that his sources of protein will probably be a lot more filling. There are also indications that calories are less efficiently absorbed from fiber-rich vegetable foods than from animal foods. On the other hand, the vegetarian who eats large amounts of cheese, peanut butter, oil, ice cream, and honey isn't doing his waist any favor. Those foods contain no fiber but lots of calories.

There is another fact about protein which is especially important to the reducer. Many people assume that when you eat slightly less food than you need to maintain your weight, everything you lose is fat. But that is not the case. A substantial but variable amount of the weight lost is actually protein. During fasting, the amount of lean tissue lost may run higher than 50 percent, and this tendency to lose lean tissue instead of fat seems to be particularly strong in older people. (In contrast, when weight is lost as a result of exercise, almost all of that loss is in the form of fat.)

If you follow the reducing approach outlined in this book, which involves eating only 300 or 400 calories a day less than you normally eat, the tendency to lose protein will be minimized. Experience, though, tells me that some people are going to overdo this somewhat, and will be losing more protein. In any case, I think it is a good idea for any person on a reducing diet to try to eat 10 to 20 grams more protein than is theoretically required. In other words, I think a woman ought to aim for 50 or 60 grams of protein rather than 40, and a man for 60 or 70 rather than 50.

What happens if you don't get enough protein? Probably the most important things that happen occur at the cellular level and you may not notice them at all, until you have an injury and discover that it's taking an unusually long time to heal. The kind of things you *do* notice may be poor growth of hair; loss of skin tone, producing a haggard look; and perhaps a general sense that you are losing your strength. When you are losing fat, the appearance of your face will change, but it will look younger. If you are losing protein, you will tend to look older, like a person who has just come out of the hospital after a long period of convalescence, which usually causes people to lose very large amounts of protein.

Protein supplements, in my opinion, are necessary only when you are fasting under the supervision of a doctor, or in cases where eating normal foods is very difficult. Chicken, turkey, fish, and lean meat have more protein per mouthful than protein tablets, and the protein they deliver is of the very highest quality, whereas some protein supplements are of marginal value. In addition, these natural foods contain important vitamins and minerals lacking in protein supplements. Brewer's yeast or primary (food) yeast are protein supplements I *would* recommend because they are really foods rather than supplements, and they contain generous amounts of vitamins, trace elements, and other valuable substances, such as Glucose Tolerance Factor, found in brewer's yeast.

At this point, I should say something about the adjectives such as "excellent" or "scant" which I have appended not only to many protein values in the table, but to vitamins and minerals as well. I have done that because I feel that the average person, in scanning a food value table, doesn't really know whether three grams of protein, for instance, is a lot or a little, or whether 600 IU of vitamin A is good, bad, or indifferent. What I've tried to do is scatter a number of these adjectives throughout the table so that in a few minutes you can easily establish some perspective in judging the significance of the values given. Like the N/C ratings, these adjectives are open to debate, but if nothing else, they are at least useful guides.

I tend to give higher adjective ratings to vegetable foods

which contain useful amounts of protein, since these foods are not ordinarily thought of as protein sources. And there is a growing amount of evidence suggesting that protein from vegetable sources is useful in keeping blood fats down, which protects the circulatory system. I've said it before, but it bears repeating here: starchy foods like potatoes, corn, and beans are *not* fattening.

Calcium. Several people who have lost large amounts of weight — 50 pounds or more — on severely restricted diets have told me that they developed chronic backaches after several months of dieting. A major reason for this is almost certainly a lack of sufficient calcium, although insufficient protein could make matters worse. Many adults drink little milk to begin with, and when going on severe diets, they often sharply reduce all dairy products except perhaps for small amounts of cottage cheese or yogurt. Beef, chicken, and fish contain extremely small amounts of calcium — at least in their flesh. Most salad greens and fruits also contain only very small amounts of calcium, and some of the calcium in greens may be difficult for your body to absorb. A number of vegetables contain useful amounts of calcium but it's unlikely that you'll eat enough of them to meet your requirements. Nutritional researchers have recently suggested that daily calcium intake should be approximately 1,200 to 1,500 milligrams a day, which is half again as much, or more, as "official" nutrition tables suggest.

The person most likely to develop a calcium deficiency is a woman past the age of 50 (after menopause, the change in hormones leads to an accelerated loss of calcium from the bones). And if that woman is dieting, or has a history of dieting, the chances of developing a calcium deficiency are extremely high. Symptoms of calcium deficiency may include aches in the middle of the back (low back pain can also be a deficiency symptom), muscle cramping and spasms, and general irritability and nervousness. The slow loss of bone density which occurs during calcium deficiency often has no symptoms at all, until, at a relatively advanced age, a fall or even a slight bump that would have been of no consequence 20 years before results in a broken hip. Osteoporosis — the medical name for the loss of bone density — can't even be detected with X rays until one-third or more of your bone mass is already lost.

Because calcium is relatively difficult to get in your daily diet, as mentioned before, I recommend that adults — particularly women — take calcium supplements to insure they are getting somewhere between 1,000 and 2,000 milligrams of this mineral every day. Still, it pays to make an effort to get calcium from your foods, too, and it's interesting that certain low-calorie foods such as broccoli offer generous amounts of this important mineral.

Iron. If the woman over 50 who is dieting is likely to develop a calcium deficiency if she isn't careful, the woman *under* 50 is more likely to develop an iron deficiency. It is the iron in hemoglobin which carries oxygen throughout our bodies, and the monthly loss of blood a woman experiences can create serious problems here. Iron deficiency can have many symptoms, but the classic deficiency is a sense of profound fatigue. Itching, skin problems, dry hair, dizziness, and other conditions you would ordinarily never associate with iron deficiency can also be produced — probably because a reduced flow of oxygen to any part of your body can interfere with whatever happens to be going on there.

Before menopause, women should ordinarily be getting about 18 milligrams of iron a day. After menopause, 10 should be sufficient. This smaller amount is also applicable to men. It's likely that most of the iron in your diet is going to come from animal foods but as you scan the table you'll notice that certain other foods, such as nuts, dried fruit, and beans have useful amounts of iron. Dairy products have virtually no iron at all. When eating a food which contains iron, particularly a vegetable food, it's an excellent idea to also eat a food which contains a goodly amount of vitamin C, because vitamin C can increase your absorption of iron from that food by 50 percent or more.

Vitamin A. A number of green leafy vegetables, fruits, and root crops such as carrots and sweet potatoes contain very high amounts of vitamin A. But in looking at the table, you'll notice that there is a tendency for many foods to have a very low amount of this vitamin while a few have a very high amount. Therefore, it's possible that even someone eating a variety of foods could fail to get enough vitamin A.

A protective daily amount of this vitamin would be anything between 5,000 and 10,000 IU.

A deficiency of vitamin A will show itself in poor adaptability to dim light, poor resistance to infection, rough, bumpy skin and slow healing of wounds.

B vitamins. This category is a combination of vitamin B_1 (thiamine), B_2 (riboflavin), and niacin. Frequently, but not always, other B vitamins such as B_6 and B_{12} are found in foods which are rich in the other B vitamins as well. In those cases where foods are particularly good in one of the three major B vitamins but not in the others, I have tried to indicate that.

Vitamin C. Vitamin C has many functions, but perhaps its most basic one is in the creation of collagen, the body's connective tissue, which one researcher has compared to the reinforcing rods in cement. A deficiency of vitamin C or an exaggerated need for this nutrient can show itself in innumerable ways, including poor resistance to infection, bleeding gums, and sores that fail to heal.

In general, it's safe to say that if you seek out foods which are rich in vitamin C, you'll be getting foods which are good for you for many other reasons as well, and are generally quite low in calories.

There are many other vitamins, minerals, and food substances which are important for your health and which I have not been able to include in this table. Vitamin E, vitamin D, magnesium, zinc, and several B-vitamin factors are chief among the missing. Nevertheless, those presented here will at least give you some idea of what you're getting in the way of nutrition for the calories in many common foods.

Caloric equivalents and remarks. These entries will allow you to compare various foods for calorie content in a very rapid way. Usually I have listed similar foods, or foods which might be eaten as substitutes. In many cases, I have also included dissimilar foods to give you some idea of the caloric relationship between "meal" foods and snack foods.

This section of the table will, I hope, be especially valuable in encouraging you to think more about your alternatives in meal planning, so that you can create meals which are very pleasing to your palate but have somewhat fewer calories than you ordinarily eat. The information will also be helpful in enabling you to analyze the caloric input of the various components of such popular combinations as a bacon-and-egg breakfast or a cheeseburger. With this knowledge, you can continue pretty much eating the kinds of dishes you want, but reduce the calorie content by manipulating selected components. You'll discover, for instance, that eating a cheeseburger without the bun will save 120 calories, while omitting the cheese instead will save almost as much — 105 calories. But you can also find out that the cheese gives you twice as much protein and six times more calcium. You'll also discover that although cashew nuts are usually thought of as being very fattening, you're probably better off serving them at a party than potato chips because each chip has the same calories as two cashews.

The remarks which I make in this section of the table allow me to offer some helpful tips — and do a little preaching as well.

Food Rating and Evaluation Table

	Amount	Calories	N/C Rating	Protein (grams)	Calcium (milligrams)	Iron (milligrams)
ALMONDS, SHELLED	½ oz. (about 11)	85	Good (if not abused)	2.6 (good)	33	0.6 (very good)
AMARANTH (cultivated *Amaranthus hypochondriacus*)						
raw greens	2 oz. (1 cup chopped)	20 (estimated)	Excellent	1.9	151	2.2
grains	1 oz.	109	Excellent	4.3 (excellent)	137	1.0
APPLES	1 medium	80	Fair	0.3 (scant)	10 (scant)	0.4 (good)
APPLE JUICE	1 glass (6 fl. oz.)	87	Poor	0.2	11	1.1 (excellent)
APPLESAUCE (sweetened)	½ cup	116	Poor	0.25 (scant)	5	0.65 (very good)
APRICOTS						
raw	3 (12 per lb.)	55	Excellent	1.1	18	0.5
dried	¼ cup	85	Excellent	2	25	2.1

Vitamin A (international units)	B Vitamins (milligrams)	Vitamin C (milligrams)	Caloric Equivalents and Remarks
0	Little	0	1 tbl. peanut butter; 3 Brazil nuts; 3 walnuts; 8 peanuts in shell; 4 dates; ½ cup milk. Main value is protein and iron. Roasting in oil increases calories only slightly. Never eat from can.
3,458 (excellent)	Scant	44 (excellent)	Cultivated amaranth greens may soon be a popular "health food," especially among home gardeners. The minerals, however, are not totally available for absorption. Similar to spinach and kale.
0	Little	Trace	Roasted amaranth grains are usually added to baked goods, or popped like corn. Good protein complement to wheat. More protein and iron than sesame seeds with one-third fewer calories.
120 (not much)	Scant	6 (fair)	¾ cup orange juice; 1 small banana; 1 large piece bread. A big apple may have 125 calories. Not as nutritious as bananas, apricots, oranges. Similar to pears.
0	Scant	2 (scant)	1 glass orange juice, 1 apple. Only value is iron. Orange juice has 45 times more vitamin C. Bereft of fiber in apple. Not recommended as beverage for adults.
50 (scant)	Scant	1.5 (scant)	1 large apple (which has 6 times more vitamin C); ½ cantaloupe with 1 oz. cottage cheese; 15 almonds. More than half the calories are from the added sugar. Unsweetened applesauce has only 50 calories per ½ cup.
2,890 (excellent)	Scant (fair niacin)	11 (good)	1 very large peach; 1 wedge honeydew; 1 small orange. A very economical source of vitamins A and C and iron. One-half cup of apricots in heavy syrup has twice the calories, half the vitamin C.
4,090	See above	5	2 peaches; 4 prunes; ¼ cup raisins. Rich in iron, vitamin A, fiber. Never eat from box or bag; enjoy with fluid like herb tea.

Food Rating and Evaluation Table

	Amount	Calories	N/C Rating	Protein (grams)	Calcium (milligrams)	Iron (milligrams)
APRICOT NECTAR	1 glass (6 fl. oz.)	107	Good (if not abused)	0.6	17	0.4
ASPARAGUS	4 medium	12	Superb	1.3	13 (scant)	0.4
AVOCADOS	½	188	Fair to Poor	2.4	11 (scant)	0.7
BACON	2 medium slices	86	Fair	3.8 (good)	2	0.5 (good)
BANANAS	1 medium	101	Good	1.3	10	0.8
BEANS, GREEN (cooked quickly)	1 cup	31	Excellent	2	63	0.8
BEANS, LIMA (cooked)	1 cup	189	Excellent	12.9 (excellent)	80	4.3
BEANS, MUNG (sprouted, raw)	1 cup	37	Supreme	4 (excellent)	20	1.4

Vitamin A (international units)	B Vitamins (milligrams)	Vitamin C (milligrams)	Caloric Equivalents and Remarks
1,790	Scant	6 (fair)	6 apricots; 1 large glass orange juice. High in vitamins but also high in fruit sugar. The whole fruit is far superior.
540 (good)	Little	16 (good)	About ¼ cup broccoli, spinach, or brussels sprouts. Almost calorie-free, they are worth their high price. Try adding raw to salads.
330 (fair)	Fair	16 (good)	1 very large cantaloupe; 5 small peaches; 2 brownies. High in fat, avocados are best eaten only on special occasions, if at all. Melons are much better.
0	Scant	0	1 very small scrambled egg; 1 lightly buttered piece whole wheat toast; ⅔ cup oatmeal. Not as high in calories as you'd think but preservatives suspected of being dangerous.
230	Scant	12 (good)	2 medium peaches; 1 fairly large apple; 6 apricots; 1 brownie. A good source of iron, better than apples, but not as good as peaches or apricots on caloric basis.
680	Good	15	¾ cup broccoli or spinach. All green vegetables can and should be eaten freely as long as they are not lavishly buttered. Use vinegar and herbs, or eat raw in salad.
480	Good	29 (excellent)	1 small cup cooked lentils; ¾ cup brown rice; 1 cup mashed potatoes. Beans aren't "fattening"—a cup of limas has 40 fewer calories than a cup of cottage cheese, much more iron and fiber.
Scant	Good	20 (excellent)	Sprouts are 89% water so you can see the rest of them is packed with vitamins, minerals, and protein. Load your salads, soups, and stews with these natural "vitamin pills." (See chapter on natural foods.)

Food Rating and Evaluation Table

	Amount	Calories	N/C Rating	Protein (grams)	Calcium (milligrams)	Iron (milligrams)
BEANS, NAVY						
cooked (other white and red beans similar)	1 cup	224	Excellent	14.8 (excellent)	95 (good)	5.1 (excellent)
with pork and sweet sauce	1 cup	311	Very Good	15.6 (excellent)	138 (very good)	4.6 (excellent)
BEEF, GROUND*						
regular	3 oz.	245	Good	21	9	2.6
lean	3 oz.	185	Very Good	23	10	3
BEEF, POT ROAST*						
lean & fat	6 oz.	490	Good (in moderation)	46	20	5.8 (excellent)
lean only	5 oz.	280	Very Good	44	20	5.4
BEEF, RIB ROAST*						
lean & fat	6 oz.	750	Poor	34	16	4.4
lean only	5.4 oz.	375	Very Good	42	18	5.4

*Note: All meat values are for cooked meat.

Vitamin A (international units)	B Vitamins (milligrams)	Vitamin C (milligrams)	Caloric Equivalents and Remarks
0	Good	0	1 hamburger (3 oz.); ⅔ cup chili con carne with beans; ½ cup macaroni and cheese; 1 cup brown rice. High in fiber, protein, and minerals.
330	Fair to Good	5	1 cup creamed chipped beef; 1½ cups cooked lentils; 2 cups cooked egg noodles; 1 peanut butter sandwich. Even with the high calories, delivers good nutrition and fills belly.
60	Excellent	0	4-plus oz. baked flounder; 2 jumbo scrambled eggs. A bun would add 120 calories; cheese, 100. Snacking on hamburgers is devastating.
20	Excellent	0	½ cup corn beef hash; 4 slices salami; 5 slices bologna, 1 hot dog. All lean beef is a good nutritional bargain but lacks fiber and vitamins A and C.
60 (scant)	Excellent (but all beef is weak in thiamine)	0	12 oz. broiled chicken; 10 oz. canned salmon; 9 oz. oil-pack tuna. This portion is average; many would eat 8 oz., some only 4.
20	Excellent	0	Represents above piece of meat trimmed of all visible fat (not internal marbling). Note huge calorie savings. Two oz. canned gravy would add about 50 calories.
140	Very Good	0	4 3-oz. lean hamburgers; 13 oz. baked flounder; 11 slices whole wheat bread. This cut of meat is loaded with fat begging to be trimmed away (see below).
36	Excellent	0	1 cup creamed chipped beef; 1 cup pork & beans in tomato souce; 1 piece chocolate cake. This cut represents about an 8-oz. serving of the above cut trimmed of fat. So although the original cut is larger, the calories are much reduced.

Food Rating and Evaluation Table

	Amount	Calories	N/C Rating	Protein (grams)	Calcium (milligrams)	Iron (milligrams)
BEEF, STEAK*						
broiled sirloin, lean & fat	6 oz.	660	Poor	40	18	5
broiled sirloin, lean only	4 oz.	230	Excellent	36	14	4.4
broiled round, lean & fat	6 oz.	440	Very Good	48	20	6
broiled round, lean only	4.8 oz.	260	Excellent	42	18	5
BEEF & VEGETABLE STEW (home recipe, lean chuck)	1 cup (about 9 oz.)	218	Excellent	15.7	29	2.9
BEEF, CORNED*	3 oz.	316	Fair to Poor	19	8	2.5
BEEF POTPIE (home recipe)	1 piece (about 7.5 oz.)	517	Fair to Poor	21.2	29	3.8
BEER: See BEVERAGES, RECREATIONAL						
BEETS (cooked)	3 (2″ diam.)	45	Fair (Poor if buttered)	1.5	21	0.75

*Note: All meat values are for cooked meat.

Vitamin A (international units)	B Vitamins (milligrams)	Vitamin C (milligrams)	Caloric Equivalents and Remarks
100	Excellent	0	10 oz. turkey potpie; 1½ grilled cheese sandwiches; 2 cups chili con carne with beans; 2 large pieces marble cake. Another fatty cut of meat.
20	Excellent	0	4 slices roast turkey; 1 cup cooked beans. This is the above cut trimmed of visible fat, which reduces the total fat by 85%, total calories 65%, size of serving 33%.
40	Excellent	0	1 cheeseburger; 8 oz. roast turkey; 12 oz. milk shake. Round steak is relatively lean so even untrimmed of fat it's not bad.
20	Excellent	0	A gram of protein here costs only 6 calories; a gram from fried chicken, 7; lean hamburger, 8; milk, 18; bacon, 22; liverwurst, 19; brownies, 95; raisins, 120.
2,400	Excellent	17	4 oz. lean sirloin; ½ cheeseburger; 4 oz. roast turkey; 10 thin pretzels. Combination of lean beef and vegetables is good; vegetables add vitamins and fiber to beef's protein. More filling than plain beef.
0	Excellent	0	Typical fatty delicatessen meat. Note that 3 times as much beef stew has one-third fewer calories. Corn beef (3 oz.) sandwich on rye with coleslaw has about 460 calories.
1,720	Excellent	6	Same quantity turkey potpie; nearly 10 oz. lean, broiled, round steak. Potpies are high in calories—but not as high as a Big Mac, with 540 calories.
30	Scant	9	1 cup cooked, diced carrots; ½ cup cooked parsnips; 1 heaping cup cooked, diced turnips. Carrots most nutritious.

Food Rating and Evaluation Table

	Amount	Calories	N/C Rating	Protein (grams)	Calcium (milligrams)	Iron (milligrams)
BEVERAGES, RECRE-ATIONAL						
beer	1 bottle (12 oz.)	151	Very Poor	1.1	18	Trace
whiskey, gin, rum, vodka, etc.	1 jigger (1½ fl. oz.)	97 (80 proof) 105 (86 proof)	Worst	0	0	0
wine, dessert (e.g., port)	1 wineglass (3½ oz.)	141	Worst	0	0	0.4
wine, table (e.g., Chablis)	1 wineglass (3½ oz.)	87	Worst	0	0	0.4
Sodas						
club	1 bottle (12 oz.)	0	Worst	0	0	0
cola	1 bottle (12 oz.)	144	Worst	0	0	0
cream	1 bottle (12 oz.)	160	Worst	0	0	0
fruit flavor	1 bottle (12 oz.)	171	Worst	0	0	0
ginger ale	1 bottle (12 oz.)	113	Worst	0	0	0
tonic (quinine)	1 bottle (12 oz.)	113	Worst	0	0	0

Vitamin A (international units)	B Vitamins (milligrams)	Vitamin C (milligrams)	Caloric Equivalents and Remarks
0	Scant (some useful niacin)	0	1 12-oz. Coke; 1½ jiggers whiskey; 1 wineglass sweet wine; 14 large cashews; 3 chocolate chip cookies; 14 potato chips; 7 thin pretzels; 2 cups buttered popcorn.
0	0	0	Many liquors once sold 86 proof are now changing to 80 proof. The caloric difference is minimal. Flavored liqueurs average 135 calories per jigger; creme de menthe or cacao, 150. Brandy and cognac same as whiskey.
0	0	0	1 bottle beer; 1 12-oz. Coke; 1¼ oz. Cheddar cheese. One glass of port wine in lieu of dessert while dining out is o.k.; sipping sweet wine every day can be very fattening.
0	0	0	A bit more than half a bottle of beer or Coke; 1 glass apple juice. Not as sweet as dessert wine, not as filling as beer, not as hard as liquor, table wine is easily abused.
0	0	0	1 bottle of cream or cherry soda has more calories than a bottle of beer. But even 1 bottle of ginger ale a day consumed as an addition to maintenance-level calories would create 8 lbs. of fat. Drinking anything except club soda with whiskey is especially dangerous for those with blood sugar problems. Very heavy soda consumption has been tentatively linked with occasional urinary irritation, even bleeding. Diet soda not recommended because of chemical sweeteners. Other caloric values (per 12-oz. serving): bitter lemon, 192; Gatorade, 60; collins mixer, 128; Dr. Pepper, 132; ginger beer, 144; Wink, 178. Fruit "crush" drinks range up to 204 calories per 12 oz.
0	0	0	
0	0	0	
0	0	0	
0	0	0	
0	0	0	

Food Rating and Evaluation Table

	Amount	Calories	N/C Rating	Protein (grams)	Calcium (milligrams)	Iron (milligrams)
BISCUITS (home recipe)	2 (2×1¼″)	206	Fair to Poor (if buttered)	4.2	68	0.8
BLUE-BERRIES						
raw	½ cup	45	Very Good	0.5	11	0.75
frozen, sweetened	½ cup	121	Fair to Poor	0.7	7	0.45
BLUEFISH (broiled or baked with butter)	6 oz.	270	Excellent	44.4	48	1.2
BOLOGNA	2 oz. (2 to 3 slices)	170	Fair to Poor	6.7	3.9	1
BOSTON BROWN BREAD	1 piece (3¼×½″)	95	Fair to Poor (with cream cheese)	2.5	41	0.9
BOUILLON	1 cube	5	Good to Poor (see remarks)	0.8	0	0
BRAN	.....	.....	.....	.....	.....	.....
BRAZIL NUTS	6 large (1 oz.)	185	Fair (if not abused)	4.1	53	1

Vitamin A (international units)	B Vitamins (milligrams)	Vitamin C (milligrams)	Caloric Equivalents and Remarks
0	Scant	0	A pat of butter on each of these 2 biscuits raises the caloric count to 278—more than 2 cupcakes and as much as a piece of marble cake. If you use buttered biscuits to sponge up gravy, you'd be better off getting the gravy with a spoon and eating cake for dessert.
75	Scant	10	½ banana or ½ a large apple; 1 chocolate chip cookie; 1 fig bar. A good dessert or snack, with useful iron and vitamin C.
35	Scant	9	2 large wedges honeydew; 25 raw cherries or ½ cup-plus of cherries in syrup. Note decline in minerals and vitamins as calories go up—typical of what food processing does.
60	Very Good	0	Curiously, has 20% fewer calories than baked flounder. Same calories as 5 oz. lean pot roast or 1 small hamburger. Fresh bluefish is one of the best-tasting of all fish; many meat lovers will enjoy its relatively robust flavor.
0	Fair	0	Ounce for ounce the same as regular hamburger, but hamburger has 3 times the protein, 2½ times the iron, more B vitamins. Bologna is about one-quarter fat.
0	Little	0	1 brownie; 2 fig bars or chocolate chip cookies. Not too bad by itself (note high iron from molasses), if spread thickly with cream cheese, calories will easily double.
0	0	0	How can you go wrong with a 5-calorie cup of hot broth? Easy—if it ignites your appetite instead of easing it. Loaded with salt.
.....	.....	.....	Bran contains calories and other nutrients but adults are not ordinarily able to digest and utilize any significant amount. Young people can absorb at least some of these nutrients. Bran cereals often have added sugar.
0	High in niacin	0	18 peanuts in shell; 9 dates. Nuts are nutritious and high in zinc, but generous snacking is ill-advised.

Food Rating and Evaluation Table

	Amount	Calories	N/C Rating	Protein (grams)	Calcium (milligrams)	Iron (milligrams)
BREADS						
Italian ("enriched")	1 medium slice (⅔ oz.)	56	Poor	1.8	4	0.4
rye	1 slice (a bit less than 1 oz.)	61	Poor	2.3	19	0.4
white ("enriched")	1 slice (1 oz.)	76	Poor	2.4	24	0.7
whole wheat	1 slice (1 oz.)	67	Good	2.6	24	0.8
BREAD STUFFING	½ cup	208	Poor	4.4	40	1
BROCCOLI (cooked stalks, cut into small pieces)	1 cup	40	Excellent	4.8	136	1.2
BRUSSELS SPROUTS (boiled)	½ cup	28	Excellent	3.3	25	0.85
BUTTER	1 pat	36	Poor	0	1	0

Vitamin A (international units)	B Vitamins (milligrams)	Vitamin C (milligrams)	Caloric Equivalents and Remarks
0	Scant	0	Ounce for ounce most breads are similar in calories. Moral: eat smaller slices. Case in point: 1 hoagie roll has 392 calories.
0	Scant	0	Rye bread is made with just one-third rye flour and is similar to white bread in nutritive value. Pumpernickel has about twice as much iron and 4 times the potassium for same calories per ounce.
0	Little	0	You may end up eating twice as much to satisfy your appetite. Not as chewy as whole wheat bread, it turns to paste when toasted and buttered, or in a sandwich with catsup. A sandwich of whole wheat bread will take longer to eat and leave you feeling more satisfied than one with white bread.
0	Good	0	Big bread eaters will save themselves a few pounds a year by eating whole wheat bread instead of white. More important, whole wheat has B vitamins and minerals not restored to "enriched" white and 8 times more fiber.
440	Little	0	1 full cup mashed potatoes made with butter; 2 biscuits (no butter). Adding gravy with fat drippings adds a lot more calories. Reserve for Thanksgiving and Christmas.
3,880	Excellent	140 (excellent)	1 dozen cooked, medium asparagus spears; 1⅓ cups green beans. Your best bet in green vegetables. It would be hard to find any food with more nutrition per calorie. Steam quickly.
405	Good to Excellent	68 (excellent)	Another fine green vegetable. Avoid drenching with butter. Try lemon juice, herbs, or adding to stews.
170	0	0	Except for vitamin A, an empty-calorie food which is 80% pure fat. A 4-oz. stick of butter has 812 calories. Try to warm butter before serving so it can be spread thinly. One less pat a day means 4 lbs. saved in a year.

Food Rating and Evaluation Table

	Amount	Calories	N/C Rating	Protein (grams)	Calcium (milligrams)	Iron (milligrams)
CABBAGE (cooked wedges)	1 cup	31	Excellent	1.7	71	0.5
CAKES						
Boston cream pie	1 small piece (see remarks)	208	Poor	6.5	46	0.3
chocolate (with icing)	1 small piece	277	Poor	3.4	53	0.8
cupcake (chocolate icing)	1 (2½″ diam.)	132	Poor	1.5	23	0.2
fruitcake	1 slice (½″ thick, about 1 oz.)	114	Poor	1.4	22	0.8
gingerbread	1 piece (3×3×2″)	371	Poor	4.4	80	2.7 (excellent)
pound cake	1 slice (1 oz.)	142	Poor (probably worst cake)	1.7	6	0.2
sponge cake	1 large piece (2-plus oz.)	196	Poor	5	20	0.8
CANDY, ASSORTED	Candy has so little nutritional value there is no point in spelling out the minor differences. Here are calorie counts for 1 oz: butterscotch, 113; caramels, 113; bittersweet chocolate, 135; milk chocolate, 147 (size of typical chocolate bar); vanilla cream, 123; chocolate fudge, 113; gum drops, 98; jelly beans, 104; marshmallows (4), 90. The grand champion is Reese's Peanut Butter Cups, one package of which, at just 1.2 ounces, has 190 calories. If you're "addicted" to candy, trying to eat smaller portions probably won't work. Better to exclude it completely.					
CANTALOUPES	½ melon	82	Excellent	1.9	38	1.1

Vitamin A (international units)	B Vitamins (milligrams)	Vitamin C (milligrams)	Caloric Equivalents and Remarks
200	Scant	41	A good way to add some bulk to meal but not as nourishing as broccoli or brussels sprouts. Avoid drenching in butter. See also COLESLAW.
140	Scant	0	4 chocolate chip cookies; ½ cup bread stuffing. Important: a "small" piece is 1/12 the cake. For a larger piece, ⅛ cake, add one-third more calories. A large piece of Boston cream pie, for example, has 311 calories.
120	Scant	0	2¾ brownies; 1 large cup ice cream. A large piece, the kind most men would eat, is 365 calories.
60	Scant	0	Equivalent to about ½ small piece chocolate cake.
40	Scant	0	1 large brownie; 1½ oz. raisins. This slice of fruitcake weighs less than half as much as the chocolate cake above. Ounce for ounce, there's not that much difference.
110	Little	0	1 large piece chocolate cake; 3 cupcakes. Topped with whipped cream, the calories hit 400.
80	Scant	0	This is a modest piece. Ounce for ounce, has more calories than chocolate cake. You might be happier making chocolate cake in loaf form and serving small slices.
300	Scant	0	Generally an especially poor choice because it doesn't satisfy a sweet tooth like other cakes.
9,240 (outstanding)	Good	90 (excellent)	Most people eat only half this much but when ½ cantaloupe has fewer calories than 1 piece of buttered toast, why stint?

Food Rating and Evaluation Table

	Amount	Calories	N/C Rating	Protein (grams)	Calcium (milligrams)	Iron (milligrams)
CARROTS						
raw	1 carrot	30	Excellent	0.8	27	0.5
cooked and sliced	½ cup	24	Excellent	0.7	26	0.45
CASABA MELON	1 wedge	38	Excellent	1.7	20	0.6
CASHEW NUTS (roasted in oil)	1 oz. (about 14 large kernels)	159	Fair (if not abused)	4.9	11	1.1
CATSUP	1 tbl.	16	Good (as condiment)	0.3	3	0.1
CAULI-FLOWER (cooked)	½ cup	14	Excellent	1.5	13	0.45
CELERY	1 large stalk	7	Excellent	0.4	16	0.1
CHEESE						
American	1 slice (1 oz.)	105	Good	6.6	198	0.3
blue or Roquefort	1 oz.	104	Fair	6.1	89	0.1
Camembert	1 oz.	85	Poor (has little calcium)	5	30	0.1

Vitamin A (international units)	B Vitamins (milligrams)	Vitamin C (milligrams)	Caloric Equivalents and Remarks
7,930 (outstanding)	Scant	6	1 small wedge cantaloupe; 2 small apricots. A great source of vitamin A and a good source of fiber.
8,140 (outstanding)	Scant	5	Serve carrots as a side vegetable with both lunch and dinner. They're inexpensive, easy to prepare, and so low in calories you can eat giant helpings.
40	Little	18	Ounce for ounce, slightly fewer calories than cantaloupe. But they are poorer in vitamins and higher in price.
30	Good for niacin	0	18 roasted almonds; 5 Brazil nuts; 15 peanuts in shell; 1½ tbl. peanut butter. Party tip: 1 potato chip has same calories as 1 cashew.
210	Scant	2	The important thing about catsup is that it has 85 fewer calories than mayonnaise and 58 less than tartar sauce per tbl. Remember when eating sandwiches and fried fish.
40	Little	35 (very good)	Another nutritious vegetable that can be eaten freely. Even when the price is high, cost of each serving is still only a few cents. Alternates are carrots, green beans, cabbage.
110	Scant	4	Although nearly calorie-free, observe whether snacking on celery calms or excites your appetite. Use generously in salads.
350	Very little	0	The blandness of American cheese makes it too easy to eat too much too fast. A bologna and cheese sandwich has 400 to 500 calories.
350	Good riboflavin	0	5 oz. milk; 1 slice American cheese. Cheese should be considered a meal food or dessert, not a snack—except for growing children.
290	Good riboflavin	0	The wedge that comes 3 to a 4-oz. box has 114 calories. When eating cheese, add 9 calories for each Wheat Thin, 22 for each Triscuit.

Food Rating and Evaluation Table

	Amount	Calories	N/C Rating	Protein (grams)	Calcium (milligrams)	Iron (milligrams)
Cheddar	1 oz. (2 small slices)	113	Good (if not abused)	7.1	213	0.3
cottage (creamed)	6 oz.	180	Excellent	23	160	0.5
Swiss	Rectangular slice (1¼ oz.)	130	Very Good	9.6	324 (outstanding)	0.3
CHERRIES, SWEET (raw)	10 cherries	47	Excellent	0.9	15	0.3
CHICKEN						
roasted, white meat only	8 oz.	413	Excellent	72	25	3
roasted, all flesh, skin, and giblets	8 oz.	549	Excellent	61.7	27	4.6
fried (including bone)	½ breast, 2 drumsticks (7.5 oz.)	335	Excellent	49	21	3.1
CHICKEN A LA KING (home recipe)	1 cup	468	Excellent	27.4	127	2.5

Vitamin A (international units)	B Vitamins (milligrams)	Vitamin C (milligrams)	Caloric Equivalents and Remarks
370	Good riboflavin	0	Best way to eat Cheddar is to melt 1 slice over vegetables.
290	Excellent riboflavin	0	1½ 8-oz. containers of plain yogurt; 9 oz. milk; ⅔ container of yogurt with sweetened fruit. Cottage cheese has 3 times as much protein as yogurt ounce for ounce but about 20% less calcium.
400	Very little	0	The most nutritious popular cheese, though Parmesan has a bit more protein and excellent riboflavin.
70	Scant	7	½ a large apple; ½ banana; 3 small apricots. Even if you go berserk eating raw cherries you can't do too much damage. But ½ cup of cherries in syrup has 104 calories.
250	Excellent (super-high in niacin)	0	4½ oz. lean and fat pot roast; 7 oz. lean hamburger. Chicken (minus fatty skin) is as economic a source of protein as lean-only round steak: about 6 calories per gram. Some people would eat less than the 8 oz. shown here.
1,790	Excellent (higher in thiamine and ribo-flavin than white)	0 (meat only)	Dark meat has only about 5% more calories than white; the difference here comes from skin and giblets. Nutrition balance better than white meat. Avoid skin but eat liver.
170	Excellent (but less than roasted)	0	Excluding bone, this is 5.3 oz. of meat, considerably less than above servings. 8 oz. of meat would have 500 calories.
1,130	Excellent	12	1 cup over 2 pieces of toast would go over 600 calories, but this is good nourishment. ½ cup over toast with fruit for dessert makes a good lunch.

Food Rating and Evaluation Table

	Amount	Calories	N/C Rating	Protein (grams)	Calcium (milligrams)	Iron (milligrams)
CHICKEN FRICASEE (home recipe)	1 cup	386	Excellent	36.7	14	2.2
CHICKEN AND NOODLES (home recipe)	1 cup	367	Very Good	22.3	26	2.2
CHILI CON CARNE (with beans)	1 cup	339	Excellent	19.1	82	4.3
CHOCOLATE: See CANDY, ASSORTED						
COCOA (in a cup of water)	1 oz.	102	Fair	5.3	167	0.5
COLESLAW (made with commercial French dressing)	1 cup	114	Poor	1.4	50	0.5
COOKIES						
assorted	6	250	Poor	2.7	19	0.4

Vitamin A (international units)	B Vitamins (milligrams)	Vitamin C (milligrams)	Caloric Equivalents and Remarks
170	Excellent	0	¾ cup chicken a la king; 6 oz. lean hamburger. Almost any way you fix chicken, the result is good nutrition.
430	Very Good	0	6 oz. lean ground beef; 7 oz. roasted white meat chicken. The noodles lower the protein density but you may find them nicely filling.
150	Very Good	0	Equal to 1 Swiss cheese sandwich or ⅔ cup chicken a la king in both protein and calories. Other caloric equivalents: 1 piece apple pie; 2 doughnuts; ¾ cup macaroni and cheese; 5 oz. lean rib roast. With ½ cup brown rice, very filling, with fewer calories than beef potpie.
10	Good riboflavin only	1	If you use milk instead of water, the calorie count goes up to about 240, making a good drink for those who wish to gain weight. The caffeine, sugar, chocolate, and milk make this a doubtful beverage for sensitive children.
130	Scant	35	½ cup potato salad; 3½ cups green beans; 1 pound plain cooked cabbage. With mayonnaise instead of French dressing, calories go up about 60 points.
42	Scant	0	For about the same calories you could have (*a*) a carton of yogurt with fruit; (*b*) a wedge of Cheddar cheese, 4 Wheat Thins, an apple, and a cup of coffee with milk; or (*c*) a bottle of beer and a dozen roasted almonds. So why eat cookies?

Food Rating and Evaluation Table

	Amount	Calories	N/C Rating	Protein (grams)	Calcium (milligrams)	Iron (milligrams)
brownies with nuts (home recipe)	1 (about 3×3×1″)	97	Poor	1.3	8	0.4
chocolate chip (home recipe)	1	51	Poor	0.6	7	0.4
fig bars	1	50	Poor	0.6	11	0.15
ginger snaps	1	29	Poor	0.4	5	0.16
macaroons	1	90	Poor	1	5	0.15
marshmallow	1	74	Poor	0.7	4	0.1
oatmeal with raisins	1	59	Poor	0.8	3	0.37
Oreo-type	1	50	Poor	0.5	3	0.07
raisin	1 biscuit-type	67	Poor	0.8	13	0.37
sugar wafers	1 large	44	Poor	0.4	0.3	0.03
vanilla wafers	1 large	19	Poor	0.2	0.2	0.02
CORN						
cooked on cob	1 ear	70	Very Good	2.5	2	0.5
canned	½ cup	70	Good	2.2	4	0.4
CRAB, DEVILED	1 cup (about 8 oz.)	451	Good	27.4	113	2.9

Vitamin A (international units)	B Vitamins (milligrams)	Vitamin C (milligrams)	Caloric Equivalents and Remarks
40	Scant	0	Brownies come in close to sugar and vanilla wafers in race for world's worst junk food.
20	Scant	0	
15	Scant	0	Fig bars sound more healthful than chocolate chip cookies, but you can see there's no real difference. The same goes for oatmeal-raisin cookies.
5	Scant	0	
0	Scant	0	
98	Scant	0	
7	Scant	0	
0	Scant	0	6 of these have as many calories as a 3-oz. lean hamburger on a bun with tomato, lettuce, and catsup. Which do you want?
38	Scant	0	If you must have cookies around the house for the kids, these would be a good choice.
13	Scant	0	Eating a sugar wafer is like eating 3 teaspoons of plain sugar.
5	Scant	0	In a dead heat with sugar wafers for the world's worst junk food.
310	Good niacin	7	½ a baked potato; 2 cups green beans; ½ small piece corn bread. Brush lightly with melted butter, or rub quickly with butter stick to reduce calories.
290	Some niacin	4	See above for equivalents. Loses B vitamins and half of vitamin C in canning process—along with taste.
0	Very Good	14	10 oz. canned salmon; 9 oz. broiled swordfish. (Some would eat about one-third less than amount of deviled crab in chart.) Plain crab has only about half the calories per oz. and more protein, but who can afford it?

Food Rating and Evaluation Table

	Amount	Calories	N/C Rating	Protein (grams)	Calcium (milligrams)	Iron (milligrams
CRACKERS						
butter	5 large	87	Poor	1.4	28	0.1
cheese (145 to the pound)	10	150	Poor	3.5	105	0.3
graham	1 large rectan- gular piece	55	Poor	1.1	6	0.2
saltines (160 to pound)	4 singles	48	Poor	1	2	0.1
cheese-peanut butter sandwiches	4 (1 packet, 1 oz.)	139	Poor	4.3	16	0.2
CRANBERRY JUICE COCKTAIL	1 glass (6 fl. oz.)	124	Fair to Poor	0.2	10	0.6
CREAM, LIGHT (See also SOUR CREAM; TOPPINGS, WHIPPED)	1 tbl.	32	Poor	0.5	15	0
CREAM, WHIPPED (from heavy whipping cream)	½ cup	209	Poor	1.3	45	Scant
	1 tbl.	27	Poor	0.15 (scant)	6	Scant

Vitamin A (international units)	B Vitamins (milligrams)	Vitamin C (milligrams)	Caloric Equivalents and Remarks
40	Scant	0	1 small brownie; 11 almonds; 1 apple; 1 glass apple juice. Not much here except calories. Eating these 5 crackers every day in addition to your maintenance calories will add 10 pounds in one year.
110	Scant	0	10 crackers weigh 1⅓ oz.—that much Cheddar has same calories but 3 times as much protein and calcium and 5 times more vitamin A.
0	Scant	0	"Graham" cracker has healthful connotations but it is basically a sugar biscuit.
0	0	0	For another 20 calories you could have a piece of whole wheat bread with your soup and get some honest nourishment while you're at it.
10	A little niacin	0	Popular vending machine item packs a surprising caloric punch, virtually same as a chocolate bar.
0	Scant	30	1½ glasses orange juice; 3 oz. cranberry sauce; 2 large peaches; 2 oranges. The orange juice has 3 times more vitamin C. Two-thirds of the calories here are from added sugar.
130	Trace	0	Using this instead of milk for your coffee adds about 20 calories per cup. Other values per tbl.—half-and-half, 20; light whipping, 45; heavy whipping, 53.
917	Some riboflavin	Scant	2 brownies; small piece Boston cream pie; 1 10-oz. glass of milk. Can easily be abused.
115	Trace	0	1 small pat of butter or margarine; 1 ginger snap; 1 marshmallow.

Food Rating and Evaluation Table

	Amount	Calories	N/C Rating	Protein (grams)	Calcium (milligrams)	Iron (milligrams
CREAM PUFF	1	303	Poor	8.5	105	0.9
CUCUMBERS (with skin)	1 small	25	Excellent	1.5	42	1.9
CUSTARD, BAKED	1 cup	305	Fair (if not abused)	14.3	297	1.1
DATES (with pits)	5	110	Poor	0.9	24	1.2
DOUGHNUTS	1 medium (3¼″ diam.)	164	Poor	1.9	17	0.6
EGGS						
hard-boiled	1 large	82	Excellent	6.5 (excellent)	27	1.2 (excellent)
scrambled	1 large	111	Excellent	7.2 (excellent)	51	1.1 (excellent)
EGGPLANT (cooked and diced)	1 cup	38	Excellent	2	22	1.2

Vitamin A (international units)	B Vitamins (milligrams)	Vitamin C (milligrams)	Caloric Equivalents and Remarks
460	Good riboflavin	0	1 heaping cup ice cream; 3 brownies; 1 medium piece chocolate cake; 2 bottles of beer—any of which would probably be more satisfying.
420	Little	19	1 carrot; 1 green pepper. You'll lose 75% of that terrific iron value if you pare the cucumber. Grow your own to avoid the wax.
930	Excellent riboflavin	1	2 glasses milk; 3 scrambled eggs; 1 cream puff. A good food for slender children and convalescents. An occasional ½ cup for adults pays for itself with protein and calcium.
20	Some niacin	0	¼ cup dried apricots; 1 oz. raisins; 14 almonds. Unless you can be satisfied eating 2 or 3 as a snack, better avoid.
30	Little	0	1 bagel; 1 piece corn bread; 1 pancake; 1 hard roll; 1 plain Danish. Just 1 a week over maintenance will add a pound in 6 months.
590	Good riboflavin	0	An egg is one of the few foods that can be boiled without losing nutrients. Protein here costs only 12.6 calories per gram (you need about 60 to 70 grams a day). By comparison, lean round steak or broiled halibut costs 6; Cheddar cheese, 16; milk, 18; white bread, 32.
690	Good riboflavin	0	This assumes addition of some butter and milk to above egg, adding about 30 calories. Even so, nutritional value is still excellent for calorie cost.
20	Good for calorie cost	6	¼ baked potato; 1 large cup cabbage; ¾ cup brussels sprouts. An excellent vegetable which tends to block absorption of cholesterol eaten at same time, as from cheese.

Food Rating and Evaluation Table

	Amount	Calories	N/C Rating	Protein (grams)	Calcium (milligrams)	Iron (milligrams
"FAST FOODS"	all "fast foods"—1 serving					
McDonald's						
hamburger		257	Good	13	63	329
cheeseburger		306	Good	16	158	2.9
Quarter-pounder, plain		418	Good	26	79	5
Quarter-pounder, with cheese		518	Good	31	251	4.6
Big Mac		540	Fair	26	175	4.3
Filet-O-Fish		402	Fair	15	105	1.8
french fries		211	Poor	3.1	10	0.5
chocolate shake		364	Poor	10.7	338	1.0
vanilla shake		323	Poor	10	346	0.2
apple pie		300	Poor	2.2	12	0.6
cherry pie		298	Poor	2.2	11.6	0.4
hot fudge sundae		290	Poor	6.2	180	0.5
Egg McMuffin		352	Fair	18	187	3.2
hot cakes with butter and syrup		472	Poor	8	154	2.4
hash-brown potatoes		130	Poor	1.3	8	Scant

Vitamin A (international units)	B Vitamins (milligrams)	Vitamin C (milligrams)	Caloric Equivalents and Remarks
			Fast foods are often high in protein, calcium, and B vitamins, but low in vitamin A, fiber, and minerals. If you eat a lot of fast foods, you should try to supplement your diet with fresh vegetables, fruits, whole grain breads and cereals, and dairy products.
231	Excellent	1.8	
372	Excellent	1.6	
164	Excellent	2.3	
683	Excellent	2.9	
327	Excellent	2.4	Same amount of meat as Quarter-pounder but lots more calories.
152	Excellent	4.2	Fish is no caloric bargain at McDonald's, thanks to sauce. Has 33% more calories than cheeseburger; less iron and protein.
Scant	Good niacin	11	
318	Good	Scant	
346	Good	Scant	
Scant	Little	2.7	
213	Some niacin	1.3	
290	Some niacin and riboflavin	Scant	
361	Good	1.6	
255	Good	Scant	
Scant	Good niacin	Scant	

Food Rating and Evaluation Table

	Amount	Calories	N/C Rating	Protein (grams)	Calcium (milligrams)	Iron (milligrams)
Kentucky Fried Chicken	all "fast foods"—1 serving					
fried chicken, mashed potatoes, coleslaw, roll:						
3-piece dinner: original		830	Fair	52	.....	.....
3-piece dinner: crispy		950	Fair	52	.....	.....
2-piece dinner: original		678	Fair	41	.....	.....
2-piece dinner: crispy		759	Fair	41	.....	.....
Burger King						
hamburger		230	Good	14	.....	.....
double hamburger		325	Good	24	.....	.....
Whopper		630	Poor	29	.....	.....
Whopper Jr.		285	Good	16	.....	.....
french fries		220	Poor	2	.....	.....
chocolate shake		365	Poor	8	.....	.....
Pizza Hut: See PIZZA						
FIGS	1 medium	40	Fair (if not abused)	0.6	18	0.3

Vitamin A (international units)	B Vitamins (milligrams)	Vitamin C (milligrams)	Caloric Equivalents and Remarks
.....	.....	.....	Rating would be "Good" except for coleslaw and rolls. "Crispy" adds 80 to 120 greasy calories but no protein.
.....	.....	.....	
.....	.....	.....	
.....	.....	.....	
.....	.....	.....	
.....	.....	.....	
.....	.....	.....	The Whopper has 300 extra calories but only 5 grams of protein more than a double hamburger at the same restaurant.
.....	.....	.....	
.....	.....	.....	
.....	.....	.....	
40	Little	1	2 dates; 1 mouthful of raisins. Slightly more nutritious than dates (per calorie) except for iron. Avoid eating from bag or carton.

Food Rating and Evaluation Table

	Amount	Calories	N/C Rating	Protein (grams)	Calcium (milligrams)	Iron (milligrams)
FISH STICKS (breaded)	6 (6 oz.)	300	Fair	28.2	18	0.6
FLOUNDER (baked with butter)	6 oz.	342	Excellent	51	42	2.4
GELATIN DESSERT (made with water)	1 cup	142	Worst	3.6	0	0
GRAPEFRUIT	½	40	Excellent	0.5	16	0.4
GRAPES, SEEDLESS	10	34	Fair	0.3	6	0.2
GRAPE JUICE (bottled)	1 glass (6 fl. oz.)	125	Poor	0.4	21	0.6
HALIBUT (broiled with butter)	6 oz.	288	Excellent	42.6	30	1.2
HONEY	1 tbl.	64	Poor	0.1	1	0.1
HONEYDEW MELON	1 small wedge (1/10 of melon)	49	Very Good	1.2	21	0.6

Vitamin A (international units)	B Vitamins (milligrams)	Vitamin C (milligrams)	Caloric Equivalents and Remarks
0	Good niacin	0	6 oz. flounder; 3 fried fish cakes. Eating with 3 tbl. tartar sauce will add another 225 calories.
0	Excellent	6	7 fish sticks; 3 large fish cakes; 7½ oz. baked bluefish; 3 oz. lean and fat broiled sirloin. Note superiority in protein and iron to fish sticks. Better yet: you can enjoy flounder with lemon instead of tartar sauce usually used on fish sticks.
0	0	0	Same as typical candy bar except candy bars are slightly more nutritious. The protein here is poorly balanced and largely useless.
10 (white) 420 (pink)	Scant	37	½ glass orange juice; ¼ cantaloupe. A good breakfast fruit. For a snack, cut whole fruit in half and slice into wedges. A glass of grapefruit juice has a dozen less calories than orange juice; vitamin C identical.
50	Scant	2	½ small apple; about a tsp. of raisins. (Raisins have a high sugar content and are too easy to eat.) A cup has 107 calories. Best nutrients iron and potassium.
0	Scant	0	A glance at the chart reveals that grape juice is basically sugar water with a good dose of iron. A glassful made from frozen concentrate has 99 calories. An easily abused beverage.
1,140	High in niacin only	0	5 oz. broiled flounder; 4-plus oz. fried oysters.
0	Trace	0	Some may find that because of the stronger taste they can use less honey to sweeten than sugar. But a tbl. of sugar has only 46 calories.
60	Some niacin	34	1 very large wedge cantaloupe; 1 large wedge casaba melon; ½ very large grapefruit. Cantaloupe has less calories, twice vitamin C, 100 times more vitamin A per calorie.

Food Rating and Evaluation Table

	Amount	Calories	N/C Rating	Protein (grams)	Calcium (milligrams)	Iron (milligrams)
ICE CREAM	1 slice or ½ cup (4 oz.)	127	Poor	3	96	0
JAMS AND PRE-SERVES	1 tbl.	54	Poor	0.1	4	0.2
KALE (boiled)	½ cup	22	Excellent	2.5	103	0.9
LAMB CHOP (lean)	2 (thick, 5.2 oz. total meat)	280	Very Good (when trimmed of fat)	42	18	3
LEMONADE (made from frozen concentrate)	1 glass (6 fl. oz.)	81	Poor	0.1	2	0.1
LENTILS (cooked)	1 cup	212	Excellent	15.6	50	4.2
LETTUCE, ICEBERG	1 wedge (⅙ of head)	12	Excellent	0.8	18	0.5
LIVER, BEEF (fried)	2 slices or 6 oz.	390	Excellent	44.8 (excellent)	18	15 (outstand-ing)
LIVERWURST (fresh)	3 oz.	265	Good	14	8	4.59

Vitamin A (international units)	B Vitamins (milligrams)	Vitamin C (milligrams)	Caloric Equivalents and Remarks
290	Some riboflavin	1	1 very small slice pizza; 1 cup buttered popcorn. Ice cream isn't the world's worst dessert—it has useful calcium and less calories than 6 thin pretzels, ⅓ cup chocolate pudding, 1 doughnut, or 1 Twinkie. All the same, keeping ice cream in the freezer can be hazardous to your hips.
0	0	0	A tbl. of sugar has 8 less calories. Buy kinds you don't really like and use very sparingly if at all.
4,565	Useful	102	Another super-nutritious, nearly calorie-free green. Some prefer it to spinach because its calcium is more available. Extraordinary vitamins A and C.
0	Very Good	0	Lamb can be a high-calorie food if you don't trim the fat. These chops, untrimmed, would total 800 calories while 6 oz. of shoulder would be 570. Lean lamb is similar to very lean beef.
10	Scant	13	1 glass orange juice; ½ cantaloupe, both of which are far superior nutritionally.
40	Good	0	1 cup cooked beans; 10 french fries. Lentils, like all legumes (e.g., peas, limas, beans) have solid protein, iron, B vitamins, fiber. They're also filling. Eat with grain product to have best protein value.
300	Scant	5	The important thing about lettuce is what you dress it with. An entire head has same calories as 1 tbl. Russian dressing.
90,780 (outstanding)	Outstanding	46 (excellent)	6½ oz. lean ground beef; 4 oz. corn beef; 8 oz. roasted white meat chicken; 8 oz. broiled halibut; 4.5 oz. liverwurst. Liver is probably the most nutritious food you could eat. Especially good for chronic dieters short on B vitamins and iron.
5,400	Outstanding	0	1 large hamburger; 2 large, lean lamb chops. Smoked liverwurst (braunschweiger) is similar. A good luncheon meat (most are poor), but avoid heavy use of mayonnaise.

Food Rating and Evaluation Table

	Amount	Calories	N/C Rating	Protein (grams)	Calcium (milligrams)	Iron (milligrams)
LOBSTER (cooked)	1 cup of pieces (about 5 oz.)	138	Excellent	27.1	9.7	1.2
MACARONI AND CHEESE	1 cup	430	Good	16.8	362	1.8
MANGOS	1	152	Good	1.6	23	0.9
MARGARINE	1 pat	36	Poor	0	1	0
MARMALADE	1 tbl.	51	Poor	0.1	7	0.1
MAYON-NAISE	1 tbl.	101	Poor	0.2	3	0.1
MILK	1 glass (6 fl. oz.)	119	Good	6.4	216	0
MOLASSES, BLACK-STRAP	1 tbl.	43	Very Good (as sweet-ener, in moder-ation)	0	137	3.2
MUFFINS, BLUE-BERRY	1	112	Fair	2.9	34	0.6

Vitamin A (international units)	B Vitamins (milligrams)	Vitamin C (milligrams)	Caloric Equivalents and Remarks
0	Good thiamine	0	Because lobster is almost fat-free it has an exceptional calorie/protein ratio: only 5 per gram. But eating with 3 tbls. drawn butter raises calories to 444 and changes ratio to 16:1. 1 cup lobster Newberg has 485 calories; 1 cup lobster salad 572.
860	Very Good	0	4 scrambled eggs; 6 oz. broiled round; 2 cups of beef and vegetable stew. 1 cup of the latter stew over ½ cup rice would save almost 100 calories, give far better nutrition (except calcium), and be just as filling.
11,090	Good	81	2 apples; 3 medium peaches. This is a high-calorie fruit with high levels of vitamins. Suitable for dessert but not as a regular snack.
170	0	0	Chemically manipulated to have same nutritional profile as butter. No advantage to the weight-conscious.
0	0	1	1 tbl. jam; 1½ pats butter. Here is an item worthy of total elimination from the diet. That 1-lb. jar in your refrigerator is 1,166 calories looking for a warm home.
40	0	0	No more nourishing than marmalade and has twice the calories. 1 cup has fat-power to add ½ lb. to your weight. Wean away from mayonnaise habit by cutting with increasing amount of catsup. Wherever possible, use yogurt instead.
263	Good riboflavin	2	4 oz. cottage cheese (which would have 3 times more protein). Overrated as a protein source, milk has outstanding calcium, but Swiss cheese has one-third more per calorie. A glass of skim milk has 66 calories; low-fat, 109; buttermilk, 66.
0	Little	0	Add to half the above glass of milk and you get more total calcium for fewer calories than from a whole glass of milk, plus a sweet taste and a good shot of iron. Contains factors which help metabolize sugar.
90	Little	0	1 piece bread with 1 pat butter; 1 biscuit. If smeared with butter, rating would drop to Poor.

Food Rating and Evaluation Table

	Amount	Calories	N/C Rating	Protein (grams)	Calcium (milligrams)	Iron (milligrams)
MUSH-ROOMS	½ cup sliced	10	Excellent	1	2	0.3
NECTAR-INES	1	88	Good	0.8	6	0.7
NOODLES	½ cup	100	Fair	3.3	8	0.7
OATMEAL (cooked)	1 cup	132	Good	4.8	22	1.4
OILS (corn, safflower, etc.)	1 tbl.	120	Poor	0	0	0
OLIVES, MISSION	5 extra large	44	Poor	0.3	25	0.4
ONIONS (sliced, raw)	¼ cup	11	Excellent	0.4	8	0.15
ORANGES						
whole	1 average size	65	Very Good	1	54	0.5
juice	1 glass (6 fl. oz.)	84	Very Good	1.3	20	.37

Vitamin A (international units)	B Vitamins (milligrams)	Vitamin C (milligrams)	Caloric Equivalents and Remarks
0	Very Good	1	Probably best way for weight-conscious to get iron and B vitamins. Although absolute amounts not in same league as meat, on calorie basis are outstanding for the nutrients. Add to soups, stews, salads.
2,280	0	18	1 very large orange; 1 apple; ¼ avocado. More vitamin A and iron than an orange but less vitamin C. Too easy to eat too many.
55	Good	0	½ cup rice; ⅔ baked potato. Best eaten without butter, as a bed for stews, meat sauces.
0	Little	0	Has only 20 calories more than 1 scrambled egg. Added milk compensates for lack of calcium, boosts vitamins A and B. Best thing about oatmeal is that it's filling. Try adding 1 tbl. bran.
0	0	0	About ¾ of a candy bar; 8 teaspoons of sugar. A small amount of vegetable oil is needed for health, but most get far more oil than required.
15	0	0	2 thin pretzels; 6 roasted almonds. A few olives as a garnish won't hurt unless you're seriously avoiding salt. But as a snack, the almonds are much better.
12	Scant	3	Why are onions an excellent condiment while olives are "poor"? For one thing, olives have 27 times more sodium (salt) than potassium; onions, 15 times more potassium than sodium. And onions—raw or cooked—help reduce high cholesterol.
260	Good niacin	66	¾ nectarine or apple; 1 very large wedge cantaloupe; ¾ of a whole grapefruit; ¾ glass of orange juice. The cantaloupe has similar vitamin C, more iron, much more vitamin A. A large navel orange has 87 calories, 105 mg. of vitamin C.
375	Good thiamine	93	A few more calories than grapefruit juice, a few less than apple juice. This portion is relatively large—in a restaurant you'd probably get 4 oz. Besides high vitamin C, oranges have good thiamine and folate, required for healthy nerves.

Food Rating and Evaluation Table

	Amount	Calories	N/C Rating	Protein (grams)	Calcium (milligrams)	Iron (milligrams)
OYSTERS, RAW	6 medium (3 oz.)	57	Excellent	7.2	81	4.8
PANCAKES (made from mix with milk and eggs)	1 (6″ diam.)	164	Fair to Poor	5.3	157	0.5
PEACHES fresh	1 (about 2½ per lb.)	58	Excellent	0.9	14	0.8
dried	5 large halves	190	Fair to Poor	2.3	35	4.4
PEANUTS (roasted in shell)	10	105	Fair (in moderation)	4.7	13	0.4
PEANUT BUTTER	1 tbl.	94	Fair (in moderation)	4	9	0.3
PEARS	1 Bartlett	100	Fair	1.1	13	0.5

Vitamin A (international units)	B Vitamins (milligrams)	Vitamin C (milligrams)	Caloric Equivalents and Remarks
270	Good	0	With 3 tbl. cocktail sauce, calorie count goes to 115, about the same as a hard dinner roll and butter. These same oysters fried have 162 calories. A cup of oyster stew has about 220 calories and excellent nutritive values.
180	Good	0	The important thing about pancakes is what you eat them with. 2 pancakes with 3 tbl. syrup and 2 pats butter are good for 580 calories. Stick to eggs and lightly buttered toast—far more protein for about 200 calories less.
2,030	Good niacin	11	¾ apple or nectarine; 1 large wedge cantaloupe. Twice the iron and vitamin C of an apple, 17 times the vitamin A—for about 20 fewer calories. But eat the same peach canned in syrup and the calorie count shoots up to about 160. Peach nectar has 90 calories per glass and only 800 units of vitamin A.
2,830	Excellent niacin	13	A highly nutritious snack for slender people. But the nutrients come at too high a caloric price for you and me.
0	Excellent niacin	0	14 almonds; 3 large walnuts; 1 large tbl. peanut butter. A nutritious snack in moderation. Always eat from shell. ½ cup salted peanuts has 421 calories. The 1-lb. bag of roasted nuts you bring home contains 1,769 calories.
0	Excellent niacin	0	3 walnuts; 2 slices salami. A peanut butter and jelly sandwich made with 3 tbl. peanut butter and 1 tbl. of jelly has 483 calories—as much as a large serving of meat. If you love peanut butter and can't help snacking on it, don't buy it.
30	Scant	7	1 large apple or nectarine. Similar to apple in nutritive value. A Bosc pear has an average 86 calories; a D'Anjou, 122. A pear canned in syrup has about 140 calories; 2 dried pear halves, 94.

Food Rating and Evaluation Table

	Amount	Calories	N/C Rating	Protein (grams)	Calcium (milligrams)	Iron (milligrams)
PEAS (cooked)	⅓ cup	41	Excellent	3	13	0.9 (excellent)
PECANS (250 or less per lb.)	10 halves	124	Poor	1.7	13	0.4
PEPPERS, GREEN	1 large	36	Excellent	2	15	1.1
PIES						
apple	1 small piece (⅛ pie)	302	Poor	2.6	9	0.4
banana custard	1 small piece (⅛ pie)	252	Poor	5.1	75	0.6
blueberry	1 small piece (⅛ pie)	286	Poor	2.8	13	0.7
cherry	1 small piece (⅛ pie)	308	The Pits	3.1	17	0.4
coconut custard	1 small piece (⅛ pie)	268	Poor	6.8	107	0.8
lemon meringue	1 small piece (⅛ pie)	268	Poor	3.9	15	0.5
mince	1 small piece (⅛ pie)	320	Poor	3	33	1.2
pecan	1 small piece (⅛ pie)	431	Poor	5.3	48	2.9

Vitamin A (international units)	B Vitamins (milligrams)	Vitamin C (milligrams)	Caloric Equivalents and Remarks
287	Excellent	10	Another excellent vegetable. Like other legumes (beans, etc.) they're high in protein and iron, but also have very good vitamin values. Good for adding bulk to stews, so you don't have to butter them.
20	Good thiamine	0	12 peanuts in shell; 4 walnuts. Probably the least nutritious of all nuts—a very poor snack item.
690	Very Good	210	Calorie for calorie, one of the most nutritious of all foods. As much iron as ½ cantaloupe, with twice the vitamin C. A stuffed pepper has 315 calories, 24 grams protein, 74 mg. vitamin C. Tip: gardeners should let some green peppers ripen to red. Vitamin A value will explode to 7,300 and vitamin C to 335. Calories increase to 51.
40	Scant	1	3 large apples; 1 heaping cup ice cream. NOTE: Pies are so caloric that dimensions are critical. A "small" piece has a 3½″ arc. For a large piece (4¾″ arc, ⅙ of pie) add one-third to calories. E.g., a large piece of apple pie has 404 calories.
290	Little	1	2½ bananas; 1 cup ice cream. A large piece has 336 calories.
40	Scant	4	3 cups raw blueberries. With 4 oz. of ice cream on top, good for 413 calories.
520	Scant	0	65 raw cherries; 6 chocolate chip cookies; 1 medium slice chocolate cake. The 45 mg. of vitamin C that would be in those 65 cherries have turned into nothing here—except sugar.
260	Good riboflavin only	0	If pie must be served, here's the one with the most protein and calcium, and some useful iron.
180	Scant	3	1 cup ice cream—which has 13 times more calcium; 25 roasted peanuts in shell.
0	Scant	1	A mince pie looks nourishing but isn't, except for the iron. It has a poorer calorie/protein ratio than brownies.
160	Some thiamine and niacin	0	Pecan pie takes the cake in the calorie department. A whole pie has 3,449 calories. 1 small piece with 4 oz. ice cream is good for 558 calories.

Food Rating and Evaluation Table

	Amount	Calories	N/C Rating	Protein (grams)	Calcium (milligrams)	Iron (milligrams)
pumpkin	1 small piece (⅛ pie)	241	Poor (except on Thanksgiving)	4.6	58	0.6
PINEAPPLE						
raw	2 slices	88	Good	0.6	28	0.8 (excellent)
canned, with syrup	2 slices	156	Poor	0.6	24	0.6
PIZZA						
homemade, with cheese topping	1 piece (⅛ of 14″ pizza; 5⅓″ arc)	153	Fair (in moderation)	7.8	144	0.7
Pizza Hut	½ 10″ pizza (3 slices)					
thin crust						
beef		490	Fair	29	.....	.....
pork		520	Fair	27	.....	.....
cheese		450	Fair	25	.....	.....
pepperoni		430	Fair	23	.....	.....
Supreme		510	Fair	27	.....	.....

Vitamin A (international units)	B Vitamins (milligrams)	Vitamin C (milligrams)	Caloric Equivalents and Remarks
2,810	Some riboflavin	0	The high vitamin A looks like a good excuse until you remember that ½ cantaloupe has 3 times as much for only 82 calories. But enjoy pumpkin pie with an easy conscience on holidays.
120	Scant	28 (excellent)	1 nectarine; ½ cantaloupe. These slices are 3½″ diam. and ¾″ thick. Some pineapples are considerably wider. Unsweetened juice has 103 calories per glass.
100	Scant	14	A good example of what happens to fruit when canned in syrup; calories double while vitamins shrink. If canned in water without sugar, calories actually decrease slightly, probably as natural sugars in raw fruit are lost. Vitamin C is also lost.
410	Good riboflavin	5	The problem with pizza is that a whole one (14″ diam.) has 1,227 calories and half of that is 614. That's not excessive if you have pizza for dinner, because it does have excellent protein, iron, and calcium. But as a late-night snack, half a pizza is brutal. Except for Pizza Supreme, one-half of a thin-crust pizza at Pizza Hut has fewer calories than a Big Mac, with comparable protein. ½ of a thick-crust pizza has from 20 to 100 more calories than thin-crust pizza. Except for scant vitamin C, these pizzas provide 25 to 40% of daily needs for nutrients listed.
.....	.....	.....	
.....	.....	.....	
.....	.....	.....	
.....	.....	.....	
.....	.....	.....	

Food Rating and Evaluation Table

	Amount	Calories	N/C Rating	Protein (grams)	Calcium (milligrams)	Iron (milligrams)
thick crust						
beef		620	Fair	38	.....	.....
pork		640	Fair	36	.....	.....
cheese		560	Fair	34	.....	.....
pepperoni		560	Fair	31	.....	.....
Supreme		640	Fair	36	.....	.....
PLUMS	1 (2⅛″ diam.)	32	Excellent	0.3	8	0.3
POPCORN, BUTTERED	2 cups	82	Poor	1.8	2	0.4
PORK*						
cured ham, lean and fat	6 oz.	490	Fair to Good	36	16	4.4
boiled ham (luncheon meat)	2 oz.	135	Fair to Good	10	6	1.6
pork chops, lean and fat	2 thick chops (3.5 oz. each)	520	Fair to Very Good (see remarks)	32	16	4.4
pork roast, lean and fat	6 oz.	620	Poor to Very Good (see remarks)	42	18	5.4
sausage	1 patty (2 oz. before cooking)	129	Poor	4.9	2	0.6

*Note: All meat values are for cooked meat.

Vitamin A (international units)	B Vitamins (milligrams)	Vitamin C (milligrams)	Caloric Equivalents and Remarks
.....	.....	.....	
.....	.....	.....	
.....	.....	.....	
.....	.....	.....	
.....	.....	.....	
160	Scant	4	½ orange; ⅓ apple. Compact size makes plums good snack items.
0	Scant	0	½ large candy bar. If you can eat 1 or 2 cups and stop, not too bad a snack, supplying a little fiber and iron. But not much better than a brownie. Without butter, I'd rate it "fair."
0	Excellent	0	6 oz. pot roast, lean and fat; 7 oz. roasted chicken. Pork is obviously nutritious but tends to be fattier than beef or chicken. Trimmed of visible fat, it's much better.
0	Excellent	0	This is enough to make a sandwich, which would have 285 calories. With mayonnaise, about 335; with cheese, 385 or more.
0	Outstanding	0	These chops contain a total of only 4.6 oz. of meat, and of that 1.5 oz. is fat. Trim all fat off these chops and you'd have only 260 calories—a 50% reduction. And the calorie/protein ratio would be as good as lean ground beef.
0	Outstanding	0	The rating would jump to "Very Good" if trimmed of fat—reducing fat from 28% to 14% and cutting calories to 350. In the same class as lean-only rib roast.
0	Good	0	A cooked sausage patty is 44% fat. You're much better off eating ham with your eggs. A small sausage link has 62 calories. 2 links, 2 eggs, 2 pieces buttered toast equals 568 calories.

Food Rating and Evaluation Table

	Amount	Calories	N/C Rating	Protein (grams)	Calcium (milligrams)	Iron (milligrams)
POTATOES						
baked	1 large ($2\frac{1}{3} \times 4\frac{3}{4}''$)	145	Very Good	4	14	1.1
french fries	10 strips (about 4″ long)	214	Poor	3.4	12	1
mashed, milk and butter added	½ cup	99	Good	2.2	25	0.4
chips	10	114	Poor	1.1	8	0.4
potato salad, made with mayonnaise and eggs	½ cup	182	Fair	3.8	24	1
PRETZELS	5 thin	117	Poor	3	7	.45
PRUNES ("softenized")	5 extra large	137	Fair to Poor	1.2	27	2.1 (excellent)
PRUNE JUICE	4 oz.	99	Fair to Poor	0.5	18	5.2 (outstanding)
PUDDING						
bread (with raisins)	½ cup	248	Fair to Poor	7.4	145	1.5

Vitamin A (international units)	B Vitamins (milligrams)	Vitamin C (milligrams)	Caloric Equivalents and Remarks
0	Excellent	31	Potatoes are practically fat-free, high in vitamins, minerals, and fiber. Learn to enjoy baked potatoes with small amount of butter or yogurt mashed in well. Also very high in potassium—3 times as much as an orange.
0	Good	16	A poor snack but not that bad a vegetable with dinner. Calorie for calorie, the nutritional profile is similar to apples. Fries from a restaurant, though, may have much less vitamin C, reducing rating to "Poor."
180	Good	10	½ cup beans or lentils. Surprisingly, has fewer calories than ½ cup applesauce and far more nutritive value. Go easy on the butter.
0	Scant	3	5 thin pretzels; ½ cup applesauce; 1 large brownie. These 10 chips weigh less than an ounce. 2 ounces have 322 calories. Basically grease and salt, with some iron.
225	Good	14	1 cup coleslaw with mayonnaise; 3 oz. hamburger patty; 1 hot dog; 1 Devil Dog. It's the mayonnaise that dilutes a good food with empty calories.
0	Scant	0	14 almonds; 10 potato chips; 1 muffin; 2 oatmeal-raisin cookies. 1 Dutch pretzel has 62 calories. Thin pretzel sticks have 23 calories per 10 sticks and twice the salt of other pretzels.
860	Good	2	⅓ cup dried apricots; 3 or 4 dried peach halves. Here's another basically nutritious food that packs too many calories and is too convenient for snacking purposes. Would be rated "Good" for nonweight-conscious.
0	Scant	3	NOTE: This is a 4-oz. glass, not 6. Higher in calories than other juices, it also has very low vitamin values, but very high iron value. Contains substance which stimulates bowels—unnaturally.
400	Good	2	1 small cup yogurt with sweetened fruit; 2 large slices Boston brown bread; 5 Oreos. A good dessert for those trying to gain weight.

Food Rating and Evaluation Table

	Amount	Calories	N/C Rating	Protein (grams)	Calcium (milligrams)	Iron (milligrams)
chocolate	½ cup	193	Poor	4.1	125	7
rice, with raisins	½ cup	194	Fair to Poor	4.8	130	0.6
tapioca cream	½ cup	111	Fair to Poor	4.2	87	0.4
PUMPKIN SEEDS	1 oz.	157	Good (in moderation)	8	14	3
RADISHES	5 medium	4	Excellent	2.5	7	0.3
RAISINS	⅓ cup (1½ oz.)	124	Poor	1.1	27	1.5
RICE						
brown	½ cup	116	Very Good	2.5	12	0.5
white ("enriched")	½ cup	112	Good	2.1	11	0.9
ROLLS AND BUNS						
hard rolls; e.g., Kaiser ("enriched")	1	156	Poor	4.9	24	1.2

Vitamin A (international units)	B Vitamins (milligrams)	Vitamin C (milligrams)	Caloric Equivalents and Remarks
195	Good riboflavin	1	½ cup rice pudding, to which it is similar except that it's completely lacking in fiber. Vanilla pudding, 142 calories, with slightly better nutritional profile.
145	Good riboflavin	0	Nutritious as desserts go but that's a lot of calories for ½ cup—much more than ½ cup of ice cream (127).
240	Scant	1	Scant ½ cup ice cream; 1 large brownie; ¼ cup chocolate pudding. Won't win any nutrition prizes but calorie for calorie is better than 3 desserts mentioned.
20	Little	0	1 oz. sunflower seeds; 1 oz. cashews; 1 cup milk. Seeds are very concentrated sources of protein, iron, trace minerals—and oil. Another "health food" that has to be eaten with control to avoid caloric excess.
0	Scant	6	Calorie for calorie, one of the most efficient foods for delivering calcium, iron, and vitamins. But because the amount we can eat is limited, only the vitamin C is significant.
15	Scant	0	The same number of calories in other dried fruits or nuts would give far more nutritive value. Iron here is good, though. A good snack for slender children. Adults can use as garnish.
0	Good	0	1 small baked potato; ½ cup beef and vegetable stew. Rice is best eaten as a "bed" for stews containing some lean meat and lots of vegetables. Brown rice is filling without being heavy.
0	Fair to Good	0	Lacks fiber and some very important trace nutrients found in brown rice but still a good food. Avoid eating drenched with butter.
0	Fair	0	2 pieces white bread. Lack of fiber and depletion of important trace nutrients makes any white bread product less than desirable. Rolls also invite use of lots of butter, sandwiches of fatty luncheon meat and mayonnaise.

Food Rating and Evaluation Table

	Amount	Calories	N/C Rating	Protein (grams)	Calcium (milligrams)	Iron (milligrams)
frankfurter or hamburger bun	1	119	Poor	3.3	30	0.8
RYE WAFERS	5	112	Fair to Poor	4.3	17	1.3
SALAD DRESSINGS						
commercial French	1 tbl.	66	Poor	0.1	2	0.1
mayonnaise	1 tbl.	101	Poor	0.2	3	0.1
SALAMI	3 slices (about 1 oz.)	135	Poor	7.2	3	1.2
SALMON						
Sockeye, canned	3 oz.	145	Excellent	17.2	220 (if you eat the bone)	1
baked, with butter	6 oz.	312	Excellent	46.2	0	1.8 (excellent)
SARDINES	1 can (drained of oil)	187	Very Good	22.1	402 (outstanding—comes from bones)	2.7 (excellent)
SAUERKRAUT	½ cup	21	Excellent	1.2	43	0.6 (good)

Vitamin A (international units)	B Vitamins (milligrams)	Vitamin C (milligrams)	Caloric Equivalents and Remarks
0	Little	0	2 rolls with hot dogs equal 590 calories.
0	Fair	0	Better than white bread (these are whole-grain wafers), but snacks should have fewer calories, more vitamins.
0	0	0	You can tell at a glance that adding more than 2 tbl. to a salad turns a low-calorie dish into a grease orgy.
40	0	0	The most caloric salad dressing. All dressings are empty-calorie condiments differing only in calories per tablespoon—Blue, 76; Italian, 83; Russian, 74; Thousand Island, 80. Low-calorie dressings average about 25 calories per tbl. If you use 2 tbl. per salad, you save 100 calories.
0	Scant	0	2 oz. boiled ham (which has more protein and iron). Salami is 38% fat and contains undesirable additives.
195	Outstanding	0	2½ oz. lean ground beef; 6 average sardines. What makes salmon so much better than the salami above? Being a natural, unprocessed food, it has only 9% fat and isn't diluted by additives.
300	Excellent	0	7 oz. bluefish; 7 oz. fried chicken. Similar in value to lean beef, but with less iron. Smoked salmon (lox) has 50 calories per oz.
200	Good	0	The reason sardines aren't "Excellent" is because of their high salt content and the tendency to eat them with mayonnaise. If you don't drain the can of oil, you have 330 calories here.
60	Scant	17	Here's something you can fill yourself on, getting good vitamin C and iron in the process. Try kraut instead of potato salad.

Food Rating and Evaluation Table

	Amount	Calories	N/C Rating	Protein (grams)	Calcium (milligrams)	Iron (milligrams)
SCALLOPS (breaded and fried)	6⅔ oz. (15 to 20 small)	367	Fair to Poor	34		See Remarks
SHRIMP (french-fried)	3 oz.	192	Fair to Poor	17.4	60	1.8
SOUPS						
commercial chicken noodle	1 cup	62	Fair	3.4	10	0.5
minestrone	1 cup	105	Very Good	4.9	37	1
vegetable beef	1 cup	78	Very Good	5.1	12	0.7
SOUR CREAM						
	1 cup	495	Poor	7	268	0.1
	1 tbl.	25	Poor	Scant	14	Scant

Vitamin A (international units)	B Vitamins (milligrams)	Vitamin C (milligrams)	Caloric Equivalents and Remarks
.....	.....	.....	Scallops are similar to lobster in that they are practically fat-free and very high in protein— and also very expensive. The problem is the breading and frying—made far worse by dipping in tartar sauce. Mineral and vitamin values for fried scallops have not been determined, but they are probably high in iron. They're also naturally high in sodium (salt).
0	Some niacin	0	If you've a yen for shrimp, eat them in a shrimp cocktail and get away with half the calories shown here. Also, remember that fried shrimp are usually served with melted butter and french fries.
50	Little niacin	0	Won't win any nutrition contests but note that it contains almost 50 calories less than 1 scrambled egg and 100 calories less than a single pancake. Also, hot soups are more satisfying than calories might suggest.
2,350	Little	0	1 slice buttered bread (the soup has twice the protein and far more vitamin A).
2,700	Little	0	1 slice unbuttered bread; ½ baked potato; 2 bites of a hot dog on bun. Bargain caloric price for high vitamin A, iron. Soup, cottage cheese, fruit makes well-balanced lunch. **Other caloric values per cup of soup** (all values for soup diluted with water per instructions; if milk is used, add 80 calories per cup): cream of asparagus, 65; beef bouillon, 31; beef noodle, 67; chicken consomme, 22; cream of chicken, 94; chicken gumbo, 55; chicken with rice, 48; chicken vegetable, 76; clam chowder (Manhattan), 81; cream of mushroom, 134; onion, 65; green pea, 130; split pea, 145; tomato, 88; turkey noodle, 79; vegetarian vegetable, 78.
1,820	Good riboflavin	2	Caloric murder as a dip base or on baked potatoes. Substituting yogurt, sour cream's twin, gives you one-fourth the calories and one-twelfth the fat for about the same amount of protein, calcium, and B vitamins.
90	Scant	Scant	

Food Rating and Evaluation Table

	Amount	Calories	N/C Rating	Protein (grams)	Calcium (milligrams)	Iron (milligrams)
SOYBEANS						
cooked	½ cup	117	Excellent	9.9	66	2.5
curd: See TOFU						
SPAGHETTI (with meatballs, tomato sauce, Parmesan cheese)	1 cup	332	Excellent	18.6	124	3.7
SPINACH (cooked)	1 cup	41	Excellent	5.4	167 (but not utilizable)	4 (usefulness limited)
SQUASH, SUMMER (boiled)	1 cup (sliced)	25	Excellent	1.6	45	0.7
SYRUPS (table blend)	1 tbl.	60	Poor	0	9	0.8
TANGER-INES	1 large	46	Good	0.8	40	0.4
TARTAR SAUCE	1 tbl.	74	Poor	0.2	3	0.1
TOFU (soybean curd)	1 piece (2½×2¾×1″)	86	Excellent	9.4	154	2.3
TOMATOES	1 (3″ diam.; 7 oz.)	40	Excellent	2	24	0.9

Vitamin A (international units)	B Vitamins (milligrams)	Vitamin C (milligrams)	Caloric Equivalents and Remarks
25	Good	0	½ cup ordinary beans; 1 cup peas. Soybeans contain valuable nutrients, like lecithin, not shown on chart.
1,590	Excellent	22	2 slices pizza; 1 small hamburger on bun. High grades in all nutritional depts. Limit bread and eat without butter. A satisfying dish.
14,580	Good	50	Traditionally valued for iron, the minerals here are largely unavailable. Best values are vitamins A and C—which are excellent. See KALE.
700	Some	18	Here's another garden vegetable you can eat your fill of. Mixes well with other vegetables and soups.
0	0	0	A good condiment for people with malnutrition and anemia—for all others, pure fat-power with a shot of iron. Avoid dishes that require syrup to be palatable.
420	Scant	31	⅔ orange; ½ apple or nectarine. Not quite as nutritious as oranges but better than apples. A decent snack but oranges may be safer—they're harder to peel.
30	0	0	¾ tbl. mayonnaise; ½-plus tbl. oil. Another high-calorie, fatty condiment. Avoid foods you can't enjoy without it—they tend to be full of fat on their own—e.g., batter-fried fish sandwiches.
0	Scant	0	1 large egg; 1½ oz. flounder; 3 oz. cottage cheese; 1½ oz. lean hamburger. Good source of calcium and iron. Excellent nonmeat source of protein.
1,640	Fair	42	½ apple; 2 beets; 1 cup broccoli; 1 wedge cantaloupe. This is larger than prepackaged tomatoes, which are not worth eating anyway. Grow them yourself to get highest vitamin content and flavor.

Food Rating and Evaluation Table

	Amount	Calories	N/C Rating	Protein (grams)	Calcium (milligrams)	Iron (milligrams)
TOMATO JUICE COCKTAIL	1 glass (6 fl. oz.)	38	Very Good	1.3	18	1.6
TOPPINGS, WHIPPED						
Cool Whip	1 tbl.	16	Poor	.....	.....	.....
Lucky Whip	1 tbl.	11	Poor	.....	.....	.....
Snow-Kist	1 tbl.	15	Poor	.....	.....	.....
D-Zerta (prepared from mix)	1 tbl.	7	Poor	.....	.....	.....
Dream Whip (prepared from mix)	1 tbl.	14	Poor	.....	.....	.....
TUNA						
canned in oil; solids and liquid	1 can (6½ oz.; chunk style)	530	Fair	44.5	11	2
same as above but drained of oil	1 can (same as above)	309	Excellent	45.2	13	3
canned in water	1 can (same as above)	234	Excellent	51.5	29	2.9
TUNA SALAD	1 cup (7.3 oz.)	349	Fair	29.9	41	2.7

Vitamin A (international units)	B Vitamins (milligrams)	Vitamin C (milligrams)	Caloric Equivalents and Remarks
1,460	Little	29	½ glass apple juice or orange juice. Much better than apple juice. Has less vitamin C than orange juice but much more iron and vitamin A. Only drawback is high sodium (salt) content. Add lemon juice and sip slowly for snack. Avoid at night; salt may cause sleeping problems.
			Most whipped toppings are lower in calories than whipped cream itself (27 per tbl.), but still rate "Poor" nutritionally.
.....	.....	.....	
.....	.....	.....	
.....	.....	.....	
.....	.....	.....	
.....	.....	.....	
170	Outstanding niacin	0	11 oz. broiled halibut; 6½ oz. ground beef. The halibut would give you twice the protein and a dozen times more A (if you could eat all 11 oz.). The beef is similar in value but has 6 times more iron. Canned tuna is very high in salt and oil. In fact, more than half the calories here are from the oil.
130	Outstanding niacin	0	6 oz. broiled halibut; 3 oz. regular ground beef. Note the caloric saving achieved by draining the oil. Adding 2 tbl. of mayonnaise would negate this saving. Tuna sandwich would have about half this much tuna.
0	Outstanding niacin	0	5 oz. broiled halibut; 3 oz. regular ground beef. Water-pack tuna has an extraordinary calorie/protein ratio of only 4.5, making it an unexcelled source of calorie-cheap protein. You'd have to eat 8 eggs (650 calories) to get all that protein.
590	Outstanding niacin	2	You can improve the rating to "Good" by going very light on the mayonnaise and adding extra tomato, onion, green peppers, carrots, bean sprouts. Celery adds bulk but no real nutrition.

Food Rating and Evaluation Table

	Amount	Calories	N/C Rating	Protein (grams)	Calcium (milligrams)	Iron (milligrams)
TURKEY (roasted, white and dark meat)	6 oz. (6 small pieces)	324	Excellent	53.6	14	3
TURNIPS (cooked, cubed)	½ cup	18	Excellent	0.6	27	0.3
VEAL*						
cutlet (medium fat)	6 oz.	370	Very Good to Excellent	46	18	5.4
roast (medium fat)	6 oz.	460	Very Good	46	20	5.8
VEGETABLE JUICE COCKTAIL	1 glass (6 fl. oz.)	31	Excellent	1.6	22	0.9
VEGETA-BLES, MIXED	½ cup	58	Excellent	2.9	23	1.2
WAFFLES (baked from mix, using egg and milk)	1 (7″ diam.)	206	Poor	6.6	179	1
WALNUTS, ENGLISH	1 oz. (about 14 small halves)	185	Poor	4.2	28	0.9
WATERCRESS	1 cup	7	Excellent	0.8	53	0.6

*Note: All meat values are for cooked meat.

Vitamin A (international units)	B Vitamins (milligrams)	Vitamin C (milligrams)	Caloric Equivalents and Remarks
0	Excellent niacin	0	Similar to chicken and lean beef. Avoid eating large portions of skin and making sandwiches with lots of mayonnaise. Use tomato to moisten. Sandwich with 3 oz. meat, whole wheat bread, 1 tsp. mayonnaise has about 325 calories—not bad.
0	Scant	17	Here's a good, starchy food you can fill up on as long as you go easy on the butter. Use cooking liquid to provide moisture instead. Who said starchy foods are fattening?
0	Very Good	0	6½ oz. lean pot roast; 7 oz. white meat chicken; 8 oz. broiled bluefish. Veal has an excellent calorie/protein ratio, and the iron in veal is especially well utilized.
0	Excellent	0	6 oz. lean and fat broiled round. You can see that veal roast is fattier than cutlets. While highly nutritious, here is a food that you can easily eat too much of.
1,270	Some niacin	16	One of the few recreational beverages that doesn't contain lots of empty calories. Try adding lemon and spices for a good snack. Only drawback is high sodium content.
4,505	Fair	8	⅓ large baked potato; ½ cup peas. Try eating a smaller meat portion and a whole cup of mixed vegetables tossed with a small amount of butter. Good vitamin A, iron.
170	Fair	0	2 scrambled eggs (which would give twice the protein); ¾ container fruit yogurt (giving 50% more calcium and two-thirds more protein). The worst thing about waffles is this: 1 waffle plus 2 pats of butter plus 3 tbl. syrup=455 calories. You might as well eat a steak.
10	Little	1	2 dozen almonds; 3 peaches. All nuts are nutritious and contain minerals not listed here—but the nourishment comes at too high a caloric price.
1,720	Scant	28	Another virtually calorie-free salad green, high in vitamins.

Food Rating and Evaluation Table

	Amount	Calories	N/C Rating	Protein (grams)	Calcium (milligrams)	Iron (milligrams)
WATER-MELON	1 large wedge (4″ thick., 8″ radius)	111	Excellent	2.1	30	2.1
WHEAT GERM (toasted, no added sugar)	6 tbl.	138	Excellent	11	18	2.5
YEAST, BREWER'S	1 tbl.	23	Outstanding	3.1	17	1.4
YOGURT, PLAIN (made with partially skim milk)	8 oz. (1 container)	113	Excellent	7.7	271	0.1

Sources:

Kaufman, William I. *Brand Name Guide to Calories and Carbohydrates.* New York: Pyramid Books, 1973.

Konishi, Frank, and Harrison, Sharon L. "Body Weight-Gain Equivalents of Selected Foods," *Journal of the American Dietetic Association* (1977): 365–68.

Kraus, Barbara, *Calories and Carbohydrates.* New York: Grosset and Dunlap, 1971.

"Nutritional Information Chart" April 1977, Pizza Hut, Inc., P.O. Box 428, Wichita, KS 67021.

USDA Handbook No. 8, *Composition of Foods.*

USDA Handbook No. 456, *Nutritive Value of American Foods in Common Units,* November, 1975.

USDA Home and Garden Bulletin No. 72, *Nutritive Value of Foods.*

WARF Institute, Inc., *Nutritional Analysis of Food Served at McDonald's Restaurants* (Oak Brook, Ill.: McDonald's System, 1977).

Vitamin A (international units)	B Vitamins (milligrams)	Vitamin C (milligrams)	Caloric Equivalents and Remarks
2,510	Fair	30	½ cup applesauce; 1 large banana; ¾ cantaloupe; 2 peaches. A good snack, rich in vitamins and potassium. If you have a tendency to overdo watermelon, cantaloupe may be more filling.
60	Excellent	6	1 large cup oatmeal; 1 jumbo scrambled egg; 1 thick slice toast with butter and jelly. Wheat germ is one health food that deserves its reputation. Especially valuable for B vitamins, iron, fiber, and trace nutrients.
0	Outstanding	0	Another special food—of special interest to the weight-conscious because it contains Glucose Tolerance Factor, which improves metabolism of sugar and tends to lower high levels of insulin (common in heavy people) and possibly decreases too-keen appetite.
150	High in riboflavin	2	1 glass (6 fl. oz.) milk; 1 oz. Cheddar cheese. Note this is plain yogurt—flavored yogurt may have 240-280 calories, the difference a result of added sugar. Try combining plain with wheat germ and fresh fruit for complete nutrition.

A Note from the Author

After you've followed some of the ideas in this book long enough to judge the results, I'd like to hear about your experiences. I'm particularly interested in learning how you personalized some of the techniques described here, or perhaps developed your own. What was most helpful in achieving success? Where were the greatest challenges? I know you'll understand that I can't answer questions, but learning about the results you obtained and the problems you had will be very helpful if we do an update of this book, and may help other people on their road to weight control. Write to me, Mark Bricklin, at "Lose Weight Naturally," Rodale Press, 33 East Minor Street, Emmaus, PA 18049.

Index

D

E

F

Q

R